NATURE'S REMEDIES

JOINT PAINS

by

Penelope Ody

SOUVENIR PRESS

First published 2001 by
Souvenir Press Ltd,
43 Great Russell Street, London WC1B 3PD

ISBN 0 285 63622 7

Typeset by Rowland Phototypesetting Ltd,
Bury St Edmunds, Suffolk

Printed in Great Britain by
The Guernsey Press Company Ltd,
Guernsey, Channel Islands

Note to Readers

The aim of this book is to provide information on the uses of herbs in the treatment to relieve joint pain. Although every care has been taken to ensure that the advice is accurate and practical, it is not intended to be a guide to self-diagnosis and self-treatment. Where health is concerned – and in particular a serious problem of any kind – it must be stressed that there is no substitute for seeking advice from a qualified medical or herbal practitioner. All persistent symptoms, of whatever nature, may have underlying causes that need, and should not be treated without, professional elucidation and evaluation.

It is therefore very important, if you are considering trying herbs for medicinal purposes, to consult your practitioner first, and if you are already taking any prescribed medication, do not stop it.

The Publisher makes no representation, express or implied, with regard to the accuracy of the information contained in this book, and legal responsibility or liability cannot be accepted by the Author or the Publisher for any errors or omissions that may be made or for any loss, damage, injury or problems suffered in any way arising from following the advice offered in these pages.

Contents

Introduction

Aching muscles and joints are given an assortment of labels in the West—arthritis, fibrositis, lumbago, myalgia—most of which are simply a medical description of the symptoms involved. Arthritis just means joint inflammation, fibrositis an inflammation of the fibrous muscle sheath while lumbago simply pinpoints the problem to the lumbar region of the back, myalgia is muscle pain.

Some of these ills, such as the sorts of arthritis common in old age, are blamed in Western medicine on 'wear and tear' of fragile joint membranes, while others may be put down to some sort of mechanical problem: too much gardening or sitting awkwardly at a desk, for example.

Orthodox medicine tends to use simple remedies to provide symptomatic relief, such as anti-inflammatories to reduce swellings or analgesics to ease pain. At times, herbal medicine can be equally symptomatic in approach, especially for the sprains and strains associated with traumatic injuries. But for chronic conditions, such as rheumatism or osteoarthritis, it takes a more holistic approach, linking many of these various twinges to the whole person and seeing them in terms of excess systemic toxins, energy imbalance or emotional disturbance.

This book looks at the various sorts of joint and muscle pains that are so common in Western society and reviews the various herbal treatments that could be appropriate, drawing on the healing traditions from both East and West as well as examining some of the many dietary approaches that are recommended.

Details of all herbs mentioned in the book will be found in Chapters 4 and 5: those most appropriate for use internally are given in Chapter 4 while Chapter 5 concentrates on those suitable for external massage treatments.

CHAPTER 1

Adopting a Herbal Approach

Complain to your GP of backache, sprains or muscular twinges and the likely remedies will be 'painkillers'—ibuprofen, aspirin, paracetamol—the familiar over-the-counter products that can be found in most domestic medicine cupboards. They are effective and speedy remedies which can rapidly alleviate the symptoms; but that in itself can be a disadvantage as it does little to treat the underlying cause of the problem.

Removing the key symptoms of pain and discomfort also gives few pointers as to true recovery: if the backache is eased by regular doses of ibuprofen, then only stopping the drug for a day or so can allow sufferers to gauge how healing is progressing. Pain is certainly unpleasant and its relief an important part of therapy, but pain does have a useful role in reminding the sufferer that a particular limb needs to be treated with a little more tender loving care than usual: sprained ankles are best not walked on, inflamed joints do not appreciate sudden violent movements. The pain helps to remind us to be more careful; take that away and the damage can soon be forgotten and easily exacerbated.

Many joint pains involve some sort of inflammation so, not surprisingly, orthodox treatments for joint pains are usually centred on use of anti-inflammatories—generally 'non-steroidal anti-inflammatory drugs' (NSAIDs). Like most allopathic medicine, this approach to therapy is aimed at combating symptoms and so reducing pain. The drugs do not aim to cure the problem or even to halt the progress of any joint disease, simply to relieve the most obvious symptom.

Table 1: Non-steroidal anti-inflammatory drugs (NSAIDs) generally used for treating joint pains.

Drug type	Example
Salicylates	soluble aspirin, enteric-coated aspirin, benorylate
Propionic acid derivatives	ibuprofen, fluribiprofen, ketoprofen, naproxen, Synflex, fenoprofen, Orudis, Alrheumal, fenbufen, tiaprofenic acid
Indenes	indomethacin, tolmetin, acetmetacin
Fenemates	mefenamic acid, flufenamic acid
Phenylbutazone	azapropazone, feprazone, Rheumox, Butacote
Phenylacetic acid derivatives	fenclofenac, diclofenac sodium, Voltarol, Motifene, Arthrotec

Problems with NSAIDs

Use of NSAIDs is not without risk and the catalogue of side effects is impressive: ibuprofen can cause colitis; indomethacin, naproxen and ketoprofen have been blamed for perforation of the colon. As well as these common gastro-intestinal problems, NSAIDs can cause kidney and liver damage, blurred vision, hair loss and may even contribute to the risk of Parkinson's disease, while Voltarol has been blamed for hepatitis and liver failure (McTaggart, 1992).

Many of the newer drugs work by inhibiting the synthesis of prostaglandins to suppress inflammation. They can also interfere with enzyme production with unknown consequences. Prostaglandins are essential for many vital bodily functions so blocking their production can trigger a catalogue of side effects with potentially disastrous results. Among their many activities, prostaglandins are essential for maintaining normal gastrointestinal activity which explains that all too common side effect of NSAIDs—digestive upsets.

According to one study (Brooks and Day, 1991), 'the gastro-intestinal effects of NSAIDs include gastric erosion, peptic ulcer formation and perforation, major upper gastro-intestinal haemor-rhage, and inflammation and change in the permeability of the intestine and lower bowel'.

The researchers found that the risk of needing hospital treatment for these sorts of gastro-intestinal disturbances were seven times as great for patients on NSAID therapy compared with patients not given these drugs. Brooks and Day added that this result suggests that '. . . in the United States, the syndrome of NSAID gastropathy accounts for at least 2,600 deaths and 20,000 hospital-isations each year in patients with rheumatoid arthritis alone'. This could be an underestimate since the Food and Drug Administration in the US estimates that the 200,000 cases of gastric bleeding each year result in up to 20,000 deaths.

Apart from these very real health risks, interfering with prosta-glandin activity to increase the permeability in the lower bowel would also allow more toxins to leak into the system—and from a herbal perspective, that could be the very reason for the problem in the first place.

Prostaglandins have an effect on the blood vessels and heart as well, and the conflicting action of NSAIDs can also increase the risk of developing congestive heart failure, especially in elderly patients. One recent study (Page and Henry, 2000) found that the use of NSAIDs (other than low doses of aspirin) could double the odds of a hospital admission for congestive heart failure and concluded that 19% of hospital admissions for the condition could be blamed directly on use of NSAIDs.

Alternative approaches to aches and pains
Herbal medicine certainly includes several remedies which can be compared with simple anti-inflammatory drugs like aspirin. White willow or meadowsweet, for example, contain very similar chemi-cals, although these are obviously in much lower concentration so

the herbs are significantly less potent than concentrated synthetic drugs. Easing pain is an important aspect of any herbal approach to treatment, but that is just part of the picture. More significant is finding the cause of the problem.

Arthritis, for example, can damage joints, but it does not just happen out of the blue; there is always some underlying cause contributing to the problem. That might be untreated joint damage or an excess of irritant chemicals in the bloodstream. And if there are irritant chemicals then how did they get there? Is it basically a dietary problem or a failure by the body to eliminate toxins from the system in the usual way? In some cases arthritis can be a direct result of food intolerance.

Case history 1: Julie M.

Lifelong joint pains linked to food intolerance

Julie M. was 43, and married without children. She sought herbal treatment for lower back pains which had been diagnosed by her GP as arthritis in the spine. She had suffered from joint pains since the age of nine when they were labelled as 'growing pains'. Over the years the pain had been a regular part of her life affecting at various times her shoulders, neck, elbows, hands and knees. She used varying doses of paracetamol to ease the pain but tried to 'put up with it' as much as possible.

Julie's mother had been severely crippled by rheumatoid arthritis and she believed that she too would suffer the same fate, although clinical tests organised by her GP had so far proved negative to rheumatoid factor and the GP had suggested the pains might be due to a lingering virus. When she persisted in trying to identify the cause of her worsening back pains she was prescribed tranquillisers.

Significantly, Julie also suffered from catarrh and was prone to chest infections with bronchitis most winters. She suffered, too, from abdominal bloating and regular digestive upsets with occasional very severe wind, and tended to feel

---

14

tired most of the time. Julie had suspected food allergy and tests had pinpointed chocolate, wheat and cheese as potential allergens. She tried to avoid chocolate and cheese as much as possible but continued to eat normal bread, not fully convinced by the postal hair allergy testing service she had used.

After the initial consultation Julie was asked to try a strictly gluten-free diet for two weeks as well as continuing to avoid chocolate and cheese. She was given a herbal tincture containing celery seed, black cohosh, meadowsweet, vervain, marigold and bladderwrack. This was aimed at cleansing the system, stimulating digestion and metabolism and combating any possible fungal infection contributing to the symptoms. She was also given a topical rub of rosemary oil in infused bladderwrack oil to use on her back, and a tea of celery and lignum vitae to drink each day.

After two weeks Julie reported that she had been pain-free for the past week and was starting to feel more energetic, although the diet was proving a problem—changing to gluten-free cookery is never easy.

Medication was continued for another month and Julie gradually found the diet less restrictive. Her sensitivity to wheat became quite apparent when two months into a gluten-free regime she indulged in a family birthday cake and woke with severe back and knee pains next morning.

Julie's problems did not totally disappear with the source of her food intolerance: her immune system had been weakened by decades of additional stress caused by the allergenic foods and she remained very prone to infections.

Her damaged joints continued to be painful, especially in damp weather. Regular doses of celery and lignum vitae tea, topical massage treatments—including infused comfrey oil to help repair the damage—plus echinacea and marigold to combat opportunist infections were continued as long-term treatments.

Herbal medicine always seeks to treat the cause rather than simply relieve symptoms. While a herbal remedy for joint pains may contain anti-inflammatories there will also be many other ingredients in the brew. Western herbalists tend to see many forms of arthritis as toxicity problems, because waste products linger in the body and eventually oxidise and damage delicate membranes. This is most obvious in gout where excess uric acid collects in joints. Treatment usually focuses on blood-cleansing herbs, diuretics and digestive stimulants with anti-inflammatory herbs to provide symptomatic relief.

These diuretics, laxatives, liver tonics or digestive stimulants will help to improve elimination, cleanse the system and remove the toxic chemicals collecting in the bloodstream and joints which might be contributing to the condition. Uric acid salts (urates)—a by-product of poor excretion—are a common problem; they can be deposited in joints resulting in painful arthritic swellings and gout. Many other toxins, by-products from nutrition or pollutants in our food, find their way into the system in the same way.

The liver is the first line of defence when it comes to absorbing the nutrients from the foods we eat, so herbalists will often treat chronic muscular or joint problems with cleansing liver herbs to restore normal function and help clear the build-up of toxins. A herbal practitioner might add yellow dock to an arthritic remedy, for example. This is a laxative which would be appropriate for a sluggish digestion, helping to speed the passage of food wastes through the bowel and so reduce any absorption of toxic chemicals which might leak back into the system. The remedy could also include burdock which is often used for skin problems such as eczema. In an arthritic treatment it would be added as a blood cleanser (depurative) similarly helping to remove toxic wastes from the bloodstream. In the past, sweat houses, hot baths and diaphoretics were also used to remove as many toxins by all possible excretion routes as quickly as possible.

Build-up of toxic chemicals can also be associated with poor blood circulation, so a herbal treatment might include circulatory stimulants, such as prickly ash, to help invigorate the system and clear toxic compounds.

Case history 2: Sarah W.

All sorts of 'rheumatic aches'

Sarah W. was 52, and had been suffering from 'rheumatic problems' since her late 20s when she had been diagnosed with arthritis affecting the spine (spondylitis). Over the years the aches and pains had continued and had at times affected her back, neck, shoulders, hips and knees as the pattern of pain shifted. There was generally a flare-up three or four times a year and she was currently taking Voltarol as need be, generally three or four tablets daily for two or three weeks until the symptoms eased again. Sarah complained she always felt cold with a tendency towards chilblains and constipation was a regular problem. She also had a weakness for chocolate bars and has been suffering from menopausal problems for the past three years.

Sarah was given an external rub containing infused bladderwrack and comfrey oils with a little rosemary, eucalyptus and juniper. Internally she was given a mixture containing angelica, black cohosh, bogbean, St John's wort and meadowsweet which would help stimulate the digestion while easing any joint inflammation; prickly ash and cinnamon twigs were added to the mix to help the circulation. Sage tea was suggested to help the ongoing menopausal problems—as would the black cohosh included in her main medicine—and Sarah was encouraged to cut down on her chocolate consumption.

Two weeks later she reported that the intermittent joint pains had started to ease, this time without recourse to Voltarol although her neck remained stiff and painful to move. She was still feeling cold and the chocolate bars had been replaced by a succession of assorted cakes and biscuits. Medication was continued for a further month with no recurrence of the joint pains.

As a maintenance therapy, Sarah was given more oils to use for her neck, she started taking courses of devil's claw tablets on a regular basis and cups of meadowsweet and vervain tea were suggested to help the digestion as well as prevent any further discomfort. Cinnamon toast and ginger tea were recommended as regular dietary additions to help the circulation.

A year later Sarah returned, this time with stress and insomnia associated with a change in family circumstances, but she had had no recurrence of the usual 'rheumatic' aches and pains. She remained free of joint pains for a further three years when a period of additional stress, poor diet and tiredness triggered a brief return to the old 'rheumatic' pattern and a need for a further course of herbal medication.

Osteoarthritis is often a problem of old age as the wear and tear on joints gradually leads to permanent damage. Long-term use of NSAIDs is the usual therapy but herbs can sometimes help to ease the symptoms just as effectively, as well as clearing systemic toxins to help prevent further damage.

Case history 3: Dorothy E.

Osteoarthritis in old age

Dorothy was an active 80-year-old, a widow with six grandchildren whom she adored and saw regularly. She had suffered from arthritic knees for five years—the result, she believed, of a bad fall 15 years previously—and in recent months her back and feet had started to ache as well. She complained of excessive tiredness and felt 'miserable and an absolute mess' with age and looming infirmity starting to interfere with her busy family and social life. She was taking more than eight paracetamol tablets a day and had found that her GP's alternative of ibuprofen led to stomach upsets.

She had recently cut out citrus fruits and plums from her diet as she had found these made the joints more uncomfortable but otherwise her diet was quite good, although she had a tendency towards constipation. Dorothy also complained that her ankles tended to swell and on examination her blood pressure (200/105 mg Hg) was rather higher than it should have been, although this had not previously been noted in her regular trips to the GP.

Dorothy was given a mixture of comfrey oil with rosemary, juniper and a couple of drops of wintergreen to use as an external massage for her knees and feet. She planned to persuade a daughter who lived nearby to massage some into her back occasionally as well.

Internal medicine was aimed at relieving the arthritic discomfort as well as stimulating digestion to improve elimination and help clear toxins from the system. It contained white willow fluid extract, celery, bogbean, angelica, and yellow dock, with St John's wort—which would also help with her low spirits—and lime flowers to help the digestion and gently ease her blood pressure, which was possibly related to her present tense mood. Siberian ginseng tablets were also given to provide a little gentle help for her stamina problems.

Three weeks later Dorothy was feeling more cheerful. The comfrey oil had provided some effective symptomatic relief and her digestion seemed to be easier. She felt she had more energy and felt less stiff in the morning, although she continued to take several paracetamol tablets each day. Her blood pressure was a more relaxed 160/85 mg Hg and remained around this level over the following months.

Medication was continued for a further two months and Dorothy reduced her paracetamol to at most two tablets daily. Her back and ankles were easier although the knee was still painful when she walked. Dorothy continued using the comfrey oil and over several months found her knee gradually improved as the old damage slowly began to heal. She switched to drinking a daily cup of meadowsweet and St John's wort tea as a long-term option. The pains in her feet and back became less constant and, importantly from her point of view, no longer prevented her from getting out and about with her grandchildren.

Like many pensioners Dorothy did not have a great deal of money to spend on herbal supplements so she much appreciated one simple and economical old remedy: crushed cabbage leaves (a potent anti-inflammatory) wrapped around her knees and ankles to cope with the occasional flare-up in symptoms after over-exertion.

At 80 her arthritic problem was not going to disappear completely, but it no longer interfered with her daily activities and she was no longer dependent on daily high doses of NSAIDs to ease her aches and pains.

While arthritis or rheumatic pains may be useful labels to describe disease syndromes each patient is very different and the associated factors contributing to the problem can vary dramatically. Poor diet, weak digestion, stress, food intolerance, old injuries, all play a part and can be tackled by subtle variations in herbal medicine. There is also the psychological dimension.

This can perhaps most easily be seen in 'frozen shoulder' where a person may be unable to raise an arm much above shoulder height. Sufferers are often men in late middle age who frequently have associated workplace stress.

Stress is a normal and necessary part of our lives: it provides a stimulus for activity and invention. Our bodies are equipped to deal with stress because our hormonal system springs into action to give us the energy for 'flight or fight' in difficult situations and the resulting adrenaline rush can provide a 'high' which is potentially addictive. Stress is part of being alive—without it we cease to function.

That 'flight or fight' response is fine if we can carry out either of these actions, but if we don't the body remains overactive, in a constant state of alertness, which adds to feelings of frustration and a sense of being overloaded. This is what is commonly labelled as 'stress' but is more accurately the 'negative stress response'. If this response gets out of hand it can also be extremely damaging for health.

There are numerous widely accepted physical symptoms of

stress and some health specialists argue that any inability to cope with stress can manifest in almost any sort of illness—from a sudden cold as an excuse to take a day off work, to an unsightly skin disease sending out a protective 'keep away' message, to life-threatening diseases like cancer and heart failure.

Rather than opting for 'flight' the frozen shoulder sufferer would prefer 'fight'—to hit out and punch the boss on the nose—but that is not acceptable in our society so the urge is repressed and the arm firmly clamped to the side, where it remains.

More severe forms of arthritis can also have this emotional dimension: the rheumatoid arthritis (RA) sufferer who finds her illness a defence against coping with the outside world and finds heavy dependence on other family members an attractive alternative to fending for herself, or those with associated psoriasis who are seeming to hold the world at arm's length avoiding emotional involvement with an unsightly skin condition that declares 'don't touch'.

Case history 4: Claire G.

Coping with personal tragedy

Claire G. was 33, married with a 6-month-old daughter. She had taught art before her marriage and planned to return to painting semi-professionally when she had more spare time. She was suffering from psoriasis and increasing stiffness and discomfort in the joints. Her knees were the worst—tender and slightly swollen—but fingers, shoulders and wrists were also stiff from time to time, although not in any symmetrical pattern. Her GP had suspected RA but blood tests had so far proved inconclusive. A great-aunt was believed to have suffered from psoriasis and her grandfather had ulcerative colitis but as far as Claire knew there was no obvious history of arthritis in the family to suggest a genetic link.

Claire was reluctant to talk about her home life beyond her evident happiness with her new baby daughter. The stiffness in her knees had started around three or four years previously, she said, and although she had occasionally had psoriasis as a teenager it too had really only become a major problem for the past three years.

Claire was given a cleansing herbal mixture for the skin problem using red clover, heartsease, yellow dock and figwort. Knees are well endowed with tendons and in traditional Chinese theory (see Chapter 3) this can suggest liver involvement. Sluggish liver performance is also a common contributory factor in skin problems so vervain and a Chinese herb called *Huai Niu Xi* were added to the mix along with white willow. She also took celery and lignum vitae in tea twice a day.

Cleavers cream was used topically on the psoriaritic patches, while bladderwrack oil with rosemary and juniper was suggested for the sore knee. Baoding balls—Chinese exercise balls (p. 50)—were provided for exercising the fingers.

A month later Claire reported that her knee was much easier and less swollen and her hands and fingers were far less stiff; the psoriasis, however, had worsened. Over the next three months Claire's condition continued to vary: the joints were generally less stiff and pain-free but the psoriasis continued—sometimes worse, sometimes better. By then Claire was becoming more relaxed and forthcoming in consultations. Eventually the whole story of how her mother had died very suddenly two days before Claire's planned wedding rather more than three years earlier emerged. The celebrations had been abruptly cancelled, the wedding when it took place some months later had been a sad, subdued affair, and Claire's psoriasis and joint pains had started soon after the honeymoon.

She had, it appeared, always been reluctant to talk about the events; remaining positive and supportive for her father and never admitting to anyone that her wedding day had been empty without her mother there. Her raw emotions were kept under control by a very 'stiff upper lip'. Perhaps, she agreed, the stiff joints and skin problem might be some physical

manifestation of this ... Claire promised to think about it all
and talk it through with her husband.

A month later the psoriasis had gone. It was three years
before Claire returned for a further consultation—she now
had a second very small daughter and needed help for some
postpartum problems—and although there had been some
psoriasis in pregnancy her joints had been trouble-free.

Taking an holistic approach to health means seeing the patient as
a whole person who is suffering not just from a set of symptoms,
such as joint pains, but from some underlying physical imbalance.
An holistic approach also means considering the emotional and
spiritual aspects of that imbalance and using the appropriate
remedies. Sometimes that can mean herbs which have these
additional dimensions, at others it may simply be time and a
sympathetic ear.

CHAPTER 2

All Sorts of Aches

There are many sorts of joint pains: from the minor and self-limiting to crippling, long-term disorders, from the acute, sudden-onset variety affecting a single limb—such as a sprained ankle or twisted wrist—to major ailments like rheumatoid arthritis which develop over many years and can lead to joint deformity and severe pain.

Arthritis is a commonly used term for a great many different disorders. Its popular use is also slightly misleading since not all joint pains are linked to inflammatory disorders. Osteoarthritis (see below), for example, is associated with joint damage and should perhaps more correctly be termed 'osteoarthrosis' to highlight the absence of an inflammatory cause for the problem.

Differentiating the causes of these various joint disorders is obviously important as treatment and general management of the problem can vary in many ways. Osteoarthritis is usually described as the 'wear and tear' variety of arthritis. Pain normally worsens with movement as the joint is damaged, so rest can ease the condition. In rheumatoid arthritis joint inflammation really is at the heart of the problem so rest can actually exacerbate stiffness and pain with patients often feeling especially immobile when they wake in the morning. Here regular movement can be beneficial— sitting for long periods at the theatre or in an airline seat will simply increase stiffness and discomfort rather than provide welcome rest.

There are many further divisions in these basic categories depending on the associated symptoms and underlying cause of the problem: the arthritis may be linked to digestive problems or it could follow some sort of infection such as mumps or German measles in adulthood. The joint pains and stiffness may be related to the menopause or could be linked to psoriasis and skin disorders. All these different types would be treated with a slightly different combination of herbs to combat the underlying problem rather than the standard anti-inflammatory and analgesic approach of orthodox medicine to relieve symptoms.

Osteoarthritis

Around 52% of all British adults suffer from osteoarthritis in one or more joints (Grennan, 1984). Incidence increases with age so that by the time we are over 65 almost three-quarters of us will be suffering from some degree of joint damage.

Osteoarthritis is defined pathologically as a loss of articular cartilage and bone damage; it can be regarded as a structural failure in the joint. The problem is not primarily an inflammatory disorder but is due to gradual 'wear and tear' (Diagram 1).

The problem can often start with accidental damage—a twisted knee or strained wrist in one's teens can lead in middle age to arthritic pains and joint problems as the injury leaves a permanent weakness in the affected joint. Obesity, too, is a major contributory cause leading to excess stress on the weight-bearing joints, notably hips and knees. Once the damage starts, biochemical changes in the surrounding cartilage can simulate overgrowth of bone cells (hyperplasia) as the body tries to correct the imbalance. This leads to further pain and discomfort as well as local inflammation as a secondary stage of the disorder.

Osteoarthritis can be associated with occupational hazards as well. Coal miners used to suffer this sort of damage in the lower back and knees, while pneumatic drill workers tend to develop the disease in their elbows.

Orthodox treatment: Generalised osteoarthritis (GOA) is regarded as a benign disease which will progress slowly. The orthodox approach is to use low-dose analgesics or NSAIDs to ease the discomfort while reassuring the patient that the problem is not serious. As the joint continues to decay, treatment may include walking aids or support collars for the neck, depending on which parts of the body are affected.

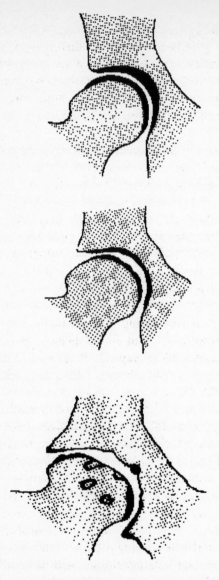

Diagram 1: Typical development of osteoarthritis of the hip: the normal structure (top) is damaged as the cartilage (centre, shown as solid shading) is eroded and there is overgrowth (osteophytes) of the bone. In advanced osteoarthritis there is further erosion of the cartilage, more bone overgrowth and cysts form in the head of the femur (bottom drawing) which will eventually cause it to collapse.

Once the decay has reached the stage where there is loss of function or as pain becomes severe, then surgery will be recommended: operations to remove loose or overgrown bones and eventually joint replacement. Hip replacements are now commonplace, although they are not always fully successful and the prosthesis generally has to be replaced every 10 to 15 years.

Herbal options: Like allopathic medicine, the herbal approach involves easing pain and discomfort but it will also seek to repair the underlying causes of the problem. Analgesic anti-inflammatories, such as meadowsweet and white willow, are often used. The initial joint damage which may have triggered the development of osteoarthritis can be helped by regular external use of comfrey oil. Comfrey helps to encourage the growth of new bone and cartilage cells and if used regularly for several months can often help to repair the damage.

Preventing further damage is also important so clearing toxins from the body and improving diet can be helpful. Calcium salts can be laid down in the joint due to dietary imbalance and small crystals of calcium hydroxyapatite have been found in damaged joints (research at St Bartholomew's Hospital, London, quoted in Bartram, 1995). This calcium build-up may be due to low levels of stomach acid which can interfere with normal calcium metabolism, so a herbalist will aim to improve digestion generally. Herbs like asafoetida, bogbean, meadowsweet and turmeric are often used for various digestive disorders as well as joint pains, while many others—such as black cohosh—are bitter-tasting, so will help to stimulate and normalise the digestion. Celery is a specific for clearing uric acid from joints so is also worth considering. Laxatives, diuretics and blood-cleansing remedies might also be included, so herbs like yellow dock or burdock might appear in the mix. Potent anti-inflammatories, such as devil's claw, could be used as well.

As well as herbal remedies there may be dietary advice (see Chapter 6) emphasising the need to cut down on foods which produce acid residues such as red meat and very acidic fruits and vegetables like spinach and strawberries. These acid foods can lead to more toxic chemicals in the joints. Eating foods which contain important chemicals to combat degenerative disorders—such as plenty of oily fish—might also be recommended.

Epsom salts (magnesium sulphate) baths last thing at night are also useful to encourage elimination of residual toxins through the skin. Several very large handfuls of crude Epsom salts (up to 1–1.5kg in total) need to be added to the bath water and the patient should soak there for up to 30 minutes, topping up the bath water with more hot water as need be. The bath should be followed with a warm shower to rinse off residual salts and then the body should be wrapped in a clean sheet before going to bed. The osmotic pressure of the Epsom salt solution absorbed in the skin encourages perspiration and draws many toxins out of the body. Moisturising lotion should be applied next morning and Epsom salt baths should not be taken by those with irritative skin disorders.

Massaging the affected joints is also useful: use dilute rosemary or juniper oil to relieve pains, while fennel and black pepper can help with elimination and the circulation.

Dietary supplements (Chapter 7) suggested could include fish oils, zinc, vitamin C, vitamin E, and selenium.

Infective Arthritis

Arthritis can also be associated with infection invading the joint. Virulent illnesses such as tuberculosis and gonorrhoea can lead to acute and severe joint inflammation.

Today these sorts of problems would be treated with high doses of antibiotics. Less dramatic infections also play a part with fungi (such a *Candida albicans*), viruses (notably German measles) and bacteria (including streptococcus, staphylococcus and *E. coli*) contributing to arthritic disorders. The joint symptoms often clear with the obvious signs of infection, but recurrence and lingering problems are not unusual. One study (Leirisalo-Repo *et al.*, 1977) of 50 patients suffering from salmonella arthritis found that in a follow-up review some months later only 20 had recovered completely while 10 had continuing mild joint symptoms and 11 had developed new acute transient arthritis. Five had acute eye inflammations linked to the infection and eight had chronic spondylarthropathy (arthritis affecting the bones of the spine).

Such causes are not always immediately apparent as the infection may seem to have cleared long before the joint problem starts: German measles and hepatitis, especially in adulthood, can leave lingering unwelcome effects. In the UK viral arthritis is found to occur in up to 35% of women suffering from German measles or 30% with hepatitis B (Grennan, 1984) leading to rheumatoid arthritis or persistent joint stiffness some time later. This sort of viral problem is less common with mumps, chickenpox, glandular fever and other virus infections.

During the acute stage, infective arthritis is usually characterised by hot, swollen and painful joints with concurrent fever and thirst. There may be an accompanying rash and general malaise. Blood tests will confirm raised white blood cell levels as the immune system combats the invading infection.

Orthodox treatment: Therapy usually focuses on relieving systems with NSAIDs and, for bacterial or fungal problems, antibiotics. With virus-related arthritic disorders treatment is simply symptomatic relief using analgesics and NSAIDs.

However, as the study by Leirisalo-Repo *et al.* (1997) demonstrated, infective arthritic problems can linger for some time.

Herbal options: Analgesic anti-inflammatory herbs, like white willow and meadowsweet, are an obvious choice but these should be supported with anti-microbial herbs, especially echinacea. For fungal problems marigold can be useful while tea tree, lemon balm and thyme oils are worth using externally.

Cleansing herbs such as red clover, cleavers, stinging nettles and burdock are also generally given alone with anti-inflammatories like devil's claw and black cohosh to ease symptoms. For arthritis associated with liver problems (such as hepatitis) then remedies which can help strengthen and protect the liver can be added: these would include herbs like milk thistle, dandelion, vervain or barberry.

Supplements of zinc and vitamin C can help boost the immune

system, while in the recovery phase immune-tonic herbs like astragalus (*Huang Qi*) or shiitake mushrooms are valuable.

Frozen Shoulder

Frozen shoulder (capsulitis of the shoulder) is a chronic stiffness of the shoulder joint associated with inflammation of the joint capsule. There is usually no obvious cause although sometimes the condition can follow injury.

Onset is usually gradual over several weeks and there is pain whenever the shoulder is moved. The condition can continue for several months or even years or may simply resolve itself quite naturally. Eventually muscle spasm fixes the joint and movement is only possible by lifting the shoulder blade and upper arm together. If untreated the condition can lead to muscle wasting around the shoulder.

Frozen shoulder can also be related to stress and tension and a suppressed desire to 'hit out' at whatever is causing the problem (see Chapter 1).

Orthodox treatment: Treatment is generally as for osteoarthritis at first with painkillers (generally NSAIDs) and physiotherapy to encourage movement. Corticosteroid injections are regularly used for persistent cases.

Herbal options: Herbalists will also approach the problem much as osteoarthritis with a mix of herbal analgesics, anti-inflammatory and cleansing remedies. If stress is a factor then relaxing nervines like skullcap, chamomile and vervain, as well as nerve tonics like St John's wort can be helpful. Siberian ginseng helps the body cope with additional stress so can be a useful supplement as well. Externally St John's wort oil with chamomile can help to ease both the inflammation and possible underlying tension.

Gout

For non-sufferers gout tends to belong in the music-hall joke category, associated with over-indulgence in port or rich food. The reality is quite different with this acutely painful disease often an inherited condition and not always afflicting those who eat or drink too much.

The pain is caused by a build-up of uric acid crystals in the joints—commonly the big toe joint. This can be associated with an inability to break down a group of chemicals called purines that are found in shellfish, red meats, and other foods. This metabolic problem may simply be due to disorders such as diabetes mellitus or obesity, but it can also, rarely, be associated with specific enzyme defects. Typically this could be a deficiency of hypoxanthine-guanine-phosphoribosyl-transferase (HGPRT) which provides negative feedback to inhibit the production of uric acid by increasing synthesis of inosine-monophosphate which in turn inhibits endogenous purine synthesis. This sort of deficiency usually presents in childhood and can be associated with mental retardation and growth defects as well as gout.

A more common cause for uric acid build-up is as a side effect to certain drug therapies, most commonly low doses of aspirin and thiazine diuretics which both interfere with excretion of uric acid by the kidneys. The increased skin production seen in psoriasis can also be a contributory cause of excess uric acid levels.

In an acute gout attack urate crystals are precipitated within the synovium and joint cavity leading to inflammation and pain. Excess levels of uric acid will not automatically trigger a gout attack; some other factor is generally needed such as joint trauma or a sudden increase in acid levels related to dietary or alcohol excess. Attacks commonly also happen at night, possibly due to different rates in water and urate absorption from joints then.

Although the big toe is most commonly the site of an acute attack of gout other joints frequently involved include the knees, wrists and foot or ankle bones.

Orthodox treatment: Drug therapy is likely to be high doses of Indomethacin or Colchicine. It is important to avoid salicylate-containing remedies with gout as in low dosages they can inhibit urate excretion. Side effects for these drugs can include diarrhoea and gastrointestinal upsets. In severe cases steroidal therapy may be used.

For long-term management, drugs which control excess uric acid levels in the system may be prescribed. These generally suppress uric acid production in the body by inhibiting the enzyme xanthine oxidase. Side effects to these drugs can include fevers, skin rashes and (rarely) hepatitis. Alternative drugs (such as probenecid and sulphinpyrazone) increase excretion of uric acid by inhibiting reabsorption in the kidneys.

Herbal options: Diet is obviously important and eliminating purines will often help to reduce symptoms as will cutting out foods rich in fruit sugars (including sweet wines and port). Foods rich in purines include: red meat, game, shellfish and molluscs, oily fish, fish roe, beans, peas, lentils and offal (especially liver and kidney). Alcohol must also be avoided as it increases synthesis of urates and inhibits their secretion. Fresh fruit and vegetables help to reduce uric acid levels—cherries are particularly good as they are rich in proanthocyanidins which neutralise uric acid.

Oxalic acid is another food residue that can build up in the joints so foods with a high oxalic acid content, such as rhubarb, sorrel and spinach, should also be avoided.

There are many traditional remedies for gout—the common and invasive garden weed, ground elder (*Aegopodium podagraria*) was once a popular gout remedy and was known as both goutweed and bishop's weed presumably because high-living mediaeval clerics were regular sufferers. Autumn crocus is a long-established anti-gout remedy although it is a potentially highly toxic herb and its use in the UK is restricted to professional practitioners only. More suitable for home use is celery seed, which can help clear excess uric acid from the system. Herbal medication is also likely to include analgesics and anti-inflammatories although the salicylate-rich herbs such as white willow and meadowsweet need to be avoided if possible. Suitable alternatives are lignum vitae, black cohosh and devil's claw. Diuretics such as yarrow or gravel root can also be useful at encouraging uric acid excretion.

Epsom salt baths (see **Osteoarthritis**, page 25) can help encourage elimination of toxins and, if the patient can bear it, topical treatments such as gently wiping with chamomile oil in a St John's wort base (or simply soaking the foot in a strong infusion of chamomile and St John's wort herbs) can also ease the discomfort.

Case history 5: Margaret B.

Suffering gout for 20 years

Margaret B. was 72, widowed with a happily married son and daughter both living reasonably close to her home. She had suffered from recurrent gout for around 20 years with the latest flare-up starting seven weeks previously. The knee was swollen and very tender and Margaret found it very difficult to walk.

She had been prescribed Adalat and a diuretic by her GP for her raised blood pressure (currently 160/100 mg Hg), but rarely bothered him about the gout, preferring over-the-counter painkillers to the prescribed alternatives. Margaret said she always felt cold and occasionally suffered from chilblains. She had rather lost interest in cooking when her husband had died a dozen years earlier and tended to eat rather too many snack foods with few fresh vegetables. She also had well-advanced Dupuytren's contracture in both hands. This is a fibrosis of the palm of the hand which meant she was unable to straighten her ring and little fingers. Margaret had become adept at concealing this deformity from her children so they would not worry or suggest surgery, which she dreaded. She had a fondness for butter which was no doubt contributing to the high lipid levels associated with Dupuytren's contracture.

Medication was focused on clearing excess uric acid and encouraging the digestive and urinary system with a combination of celery seeds, dandelion, yarrow and angelica. Prickly ash and cinnamon twigs were added to help with the circulation. A diet sheet detailed the foods to avoid.

Two weeks later the gouty flare-up had cleared but she complained of pain and stiffness in her neck and shoulders, her ankles and feet ached and walking was still an effort;

---

moreover Margaret still felt very cold. Medication was continued with more emphasis on the black cohosh and digestive stimulants such as vervain and yellow dock added. She was given a massage rub containing rosemary, juniper and infused comfrey oils.

Treatment continued with few changes for two months during which time Margaret began once more to walk regularly to her local shops as she tried to regain an interest in cooking to improve her rather inadequate diet. Three months after starting herbal treatment she was feeling much more energetic, there had been no recurrence of the gout and her other vague joint and muscle pains had cleared.

Margaret decided to try herbal alternatives for her blood pressure and this was eventually brought under control by herbal teas quite satisfactorily without the need for more prescription drugs. The gout reappeared a couple of times over the years but celery seed tea and a return to a more careful diet quickly solved the problem. When she was 82 she fell and broke her hip while shopping and never fully recovered. She died from a stroke a few weeks later.

Rheumatoid Arthritis

Rheumatoid arthritis (RA) is a chronic inflammatory disorder generally affecting the synovium leading to destruction of cartilage (see Diagram 2).

The exact cause is uncertain although it can sometimes be triggered by stress, food intolerance or infection and there is often genetic disposition to the illness. One study suggests that it can be caused by the antibodies formed to combat the micro-organisms responsible for cystitis, which some argue could explain why RA is more common in women since they are most likely to suffer from cystitis (Ebringer, 1991). Rheumatoid arthritis is also classified as an auto-immune disease where the body apparently turns on itself to destroy healthy tissue.

According to one herbalist's analysis of a number of case

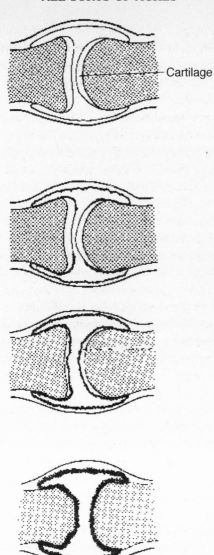

Cartilage

Diagram 2: Typical development of rheumatoid arthritis in a small joint: the normal structure (top) has a healthy synovium which becomes inflamed (second from top) and starts to damage the cartilage around the bone. This leads eventually to total loss of cartilage and eventually bone erosion (bottom drawing).

histories (Zeylstra, 1991) other predisposing factors include an inability to sweat, a tendency to suffer from chronic constipation, obesity, poor circulation, and a tendency to high blood pressure. Onset can also coincide with the menopause and sufferers tend to be susceptible to cold, with symptoms generally worse in the winter than summer. As with other sorts of arthritis these factors suggest that poor elimination can be part of the problem.

RA can affect any part of the body but will typically start with the joints of the hands, wrists and feet and progression is usually symmetrical so that both sets of fingers or both knees will be affected together. Onset is generally gradual although it can be quite sudden, especially in young people. It usually starts with general weakness, tiredness, stiffness in specific joints and vague joint pains and then progresses to painful, hot, swollen joints which can become permanently deformed in the process.

Orthodox treatment: As with other forms of arthritis the standard approach is to use anti-inflammatories—generally starting with aspirin and ibuprofen and progressing through the range of NSAIDs. Chrysotherapy, using gold-based preparations like Myocrisin, is also used for treating RA although side effects can be a problem; as with D-penicillamine treatments—another common therapy used for severe cases. Side effects of these drugs can include rashes, mouth ulcers and blood cell irregularities. Stronger anti-inflammatories, such as corticosteroids, are used in rare cases but have even more significant side effects (including Cushing's syndrome and osteoporosis); immune-suppressant remedies, such as cyclophosphamide, are used in severe cases which do not respond to other treatments.

A recent approach has been to focus on the immune issue. Researchers at University College, London (Matthews, 2000) believe they have discovered that the body's immune system turns on itself because the B-cells in the blood (a type of white blood cell involved in the immune system) accidentally create the wrong sort of antibodies and it is these which then turn on healthy joints. Unfortunately once the production of these rogue antibodies is triggered, the B-cells will then continue to produce them indefinitely. 'It probably takes just one genetic mistake in a lifetime to trigger this reaction,' says Professor Jonathan Edwards, leader of the UCL research team, 'but once it gets going it becomes a vicious circle.'

The research team has found that using drugs which seek out and destroy B-cells this cycle can be broken. When fresh B-cells are produced the chances of making the same genetic mistake as their predecessors are slim, and the auto-immune attack ceases.

In pilot tests the first five patients given the anti-B-cell treatment were almost pain-free within 18 months with the lingering discomfort due to residual damage in the joints rather than continuing inflammatory disease. Of 20 patients studied in the early trials only two found no benefit from the treatment.

Although it could be several more years before this sort of therapy becomes generally available the researchers are optimistic that it could prove beneficial for many of the UK's estimated 750,000 RA sufferers.

Herbal options: As with other forms of arthritis, the herbal approach tends to focus on clearing toxins from the system, reducing inflammation and easing symptoms in an effort to prevent further joint damage. Elimination of toxins is encouraged with diuretics, digestive stimulants and diaphoretic herbs to encourage excretion via urine, bowels and skin. Among diuretic remedies commonly used are dandelion leaf, celery seed, parsley seed and birch leaf, which is able to encourage the excretion of excess sodium salts such as monosodium urate.

Chronic constipation can often be a problem in RA so herbs like psyllium seed, which acts as a bulking laxative, and cramp bark, which helps to relax the smooth muscles of the gut, are also effective. More stimulating laxatives, such as yellow dock, can be helpful but should only be used in moderation to help kick-start the system and avoid the excess gut irritation they can cause with long-term use.

Diet is important in RA. Many sufferers find it difficult to prepare food so they tend to exist on pre-prepared meals and convenience food. Dried fruits, such as figs, prunes and apricots, all help improve bowel motions and are comparatively easy to add to the existing diet. Increasing fresh fruit and vegetable intake is also essential.

Among suitable diaphoretics to encourage sweating and further elimination of toxins are elderflower, lime flowers and yarrow which can be combined and taken in teas. Epsom salt baths (see **Osteoarthritis**, page 25) can help as well. These should be repeated once a fortnight until the level of toxins drawn from the skin by such treatments (as seen by discolouration on the sheets) is significantly reduced.

As well as poor elimination, poor circulation is a common factor so the herbal medicine will include circulatory stimulants such as prickly ash or cinnamon twigs. Heart tonics and blood pressure remedies—typically hawthorn or cramp bark—can also be appropriate while rutin extracts or buckwheat can help improve the quality of the arteries themselves. Lime flowers, garlic or ginkgo can be appropriate too if there is any athero-sclerosis (hardening of the arteries) adding to the circulation problems.

The herbal analgesic anti-inflammatories, such as white willow and meadowsweet, are almost always included in RA remedies. Many herbalists also find that white bryony is very effective, although this is a potent herb and not really suitable for home use.

Stinging nettle, too, can be helpful as it is anti-allergenic so can help to reduce the strains on the immune system. It is also diuretic and a gentle metabolic stimulant although more recent studies (see Chapter 4) suggest that it could enhance the effect of anti-inflammatory remedies as well.

Feverfew is a popular RA remedy to ease pain, and externally, herbalists may also use nettle juice, yellow jasmine or monkshood tinctures. These last two herbs are restricted for practitioner-use only, so for home use dilute rosemary or pine oils, cold ice packs, or wintergreen liniment may be more accessible.

A psychological dimension to RA often occurs: RA patients can be self-centred and enjoy the attention their condition demands.

Many women sufferers have highly attentive husbands and the illness can seem to act as a further encouragement for dependence. Obviously not all sufferers come into this category but it can be a significant factor militating against any will to recover and needs careful and sensitive handling on the part of the practitioner. Bach flower remedies such as chicory, which helps to combat possessiveness and self-pity, or heather, for excessive self-centredness, can be helpful here.

Case history 6: Jennifer W.

Sudden onset RA in an over-busy life

Jennifer W. was 34, married with two children aged seven and 11 and working full-time running her own hairdressing salon. Six months previously she had suddenly experienced severe stiffness, swelling and pain in her hands and feet and hospital tests had confirmed rheumatoid arthritis. She regularly suffered from conjunctivitis and vaginal thrush, always felt cold and was exhausted by the demands of family, work and illness. She admitted that her diet was fairly awful as her children would only eat junk food and she had no time to prepare proper meals so everyone ate convenience food. Her GP was currently experimenting with various NSAIDs to find which was most effective.

She was given a herbal mixture containing echinacea and marigold to combat underlying infections; white willow and black cohosh, to help combat the joint inflammation; yellow dock and vervain for the digestion, and skullcap to try and calm her obvious anxiety and nervous tension. Diet was discussed and simple but practical improvements she could make were advised—she promised to 'try harder' with fresh fruits and vegetables.

Herbal medication continued over the next six months while her arthritic symptoms waxed and waned, as did her NSAID medication. Diet gradually improved, but she still suffered from recurrent infections so the echinacea was supported with astragalus (*Huang Qi*). Celery and lignum vitae tea proved very effective at easing the ongoing inflammation and her initial concerns about such a potentially crippling health problem began to recede.

Her fingers and hands were most severely affected, which tended to interfere with her work as a hairdresser, while she found that many of the hairsprays she needed to use seemed to exacerbate her recurrent conjunctivitis. Significantly, whenever Jennifer went on holiday for a week she would be totally symptom-free. Her GP suggested the RA was related to some underlying virus and it was worse whenever she had a cold or felt run-down and exhausted. Eventually Jennifer took a partner into the business and was able to cut down on her hours. She improved dramatically and a couple of months later regular hospital tests confirmed a sharp reduction in rheumatoid symptoms; she stopped all medication.

Three years later Jennifer was back. Her husband's business had prospered and she had given up work. There had been no recurrence of any arthritis—but could herbs please do something for her PMT?

Juvenile-onset Arthritis

There are various forms of chronic arthritis in childhood, which by definition start before age 16 and last for at least three months. Around one child in 2,000 is affected: in some cases these illnesses develop into ankylosing spondylitis or rheumatoid arthritis in adulthood, although more commonly they do not. The illness can be associated with infection—bacterial or viral—and there may be associated blood disorders, including anaemia. Orthodox treatment usually focuses on NSAIDs with some corticosteroidal treatment in acute phases.

Children usually 'grow out' of the problem eventually, although they may be left with a joint stiffness and a tendency to arthritis in later life.

There is some evidence that the problem is psychosomatic in

origin and may be associated with broken homes or bereavement with subsequent disruption to family life. Indeed, anecdotal evidence from practitioners suggests that few sufferers come from balanced, happy family environments.

Orthodox treatment: Drug treatment usually centres on NSAIDs, although steroidal therapy is sometimes used in acute phases for short periods. Other options tend to be as for RA. Splints are also used to try to prevent too much deformity to young growing joints and most children are also given physiotherapy and exercise programmes to combat muscle wasting.

Herbal options: Herbal therapy is likely to include relaxing nervines and remedies to combat stress as well as anti-inflammatories and cleansing remedies. Typical remedies can include white willow, white poplar, black cohosh or bogbean to combat the inflammation and pain along with stinging nettles or yarrow to help with cleansing the system and chamomile, skullcap or passion flower to ease nervous tensions.

Externally hot poultices of slippery elm (a drawing remedy for toxins) and gentle rubbing with dilute chamomile oil or infused St John's wort oil can also help. Children's joints should not be vigorously massaged but given only gentle passive manipulation.

Digestion-Related Arthritis

Some sorts of arthritis are seen as digestion-related—either as an aspect of food intolerance (see Chapter 1) or linked to bowel disorders. There is also a genetic link between some bowel disorders such as ulcerative colitis and Crohn's disease and a tendency to rheumatoid arthritis or ankylosing spondylitis. In many cases the arthritic problems seem to disappear once the bowel disorder clears up.

Around 20% of men suffering from ankylosing spondylitis also have ulcerative colitis, while almost a third of those suffering from Crohn's disease also have either some form of peripheral arthritis or ankylosing spondylitis. These disorders are included in a group of genetically related illnesses called seronegative arthropathies which also includes iritis (eye inflammation), psoriatic arthritis and Reiter's syndrome (a combination of conjunctivitis, arthritis and urethritis).

Chronic bowel conditions like ulcerative colitis and Crohn's disease can cause heavy drainage of vitamins and minerals from the body and calcium may even be leached from the bones to restore blood calcium levels; this can lead to more severe bone damage if left untreated.

Orthodox treatment: Again, treatment will centre on NSAIDs although use of corticosteroids is also common for both Crohn's disease and ulcerative colitis. Surgery too is an option with total proctocolectomy in severe cases of ulcerative colitis or bowel resection in Crohn's disease. Other options for ulcerative colitis include steroid enemas and use of immune-suppressant drugs.

Herbal options: For the herbalist, the main emphasis will be on the bowel problem using soothing and strengthening digestive herbs such as fenugreek, wild yam, lemon balm, sweet flag, agrimony or golden seal. Meadowsweet, which is useful for both bowel and arthritic problems, is an obvious choice as well.

Once the bowel problems begin to ease, the arthritis usually does too, and treatment can then focus on any lingering joint problems associated with residual damage much as for osteoarthritis.

Ankylosing Spondylitis
This is an inflammatory disease affecting the bones of the spine and is usually found in young adults with men more likely to be affected than women. There is a genetic predisposition with the disease often associated with other seronegative arthropathies (see above).The problem generally starts in the lower back (the lumbar region) or the sacroiliac joint and can progress up the spine to reach the cervical region in severe cases (Diagram 3). As with RA there is inflammation of the synovium to bone abnormalities damaging the vertebrae.

Symptoms generally start with pain in the lower back and

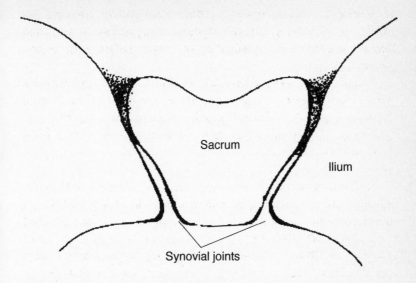

Diagram 3: The sacroiliac joints: in ankylosing spondylitis early inflammation often occurs here, in the synovial joints.

buttocks which can radiate to the thighs. Stiffness is usually worse in the morning and at rest and is relieved by walking about. As the thoracic or cervical regions become affected it can become painful to breathe. The spine can become fragile in the advanced stages of the illness, with a high risk of fracture.

Orthodox treatment: This is broadly similar to therapies used for RA starting with NSAIDs and progressing in severe cases to corticosteroids, although the disease-suppressing drugs used for RA (such as gold and penicillamine) have little effect. Exercise and physiotherapy are important to limit spinal damage.

Herbal options: Treatment is very similar to the approach adopted for rheumatoid arthritis, using anti-inflammatories and analgesics such as white willow, devil's claw or lignum vitae. The sort of cleansing regime suggested for RA can be helpful and massage with lavender or rosemary can help ease the discomfort. Topical muscle relaxants, such as cramp bark, black cohosh or lobelia tincture, can also ease the pain and can be used in compresses.

Menopausal Arthritis
Joint stiffness can also occur at the menopause when it is related to reduced output of progesterone and oestrogen. This is usually classified as a variant of rheumatoid arthritis which often appears to start at the menopause.

Orthodox treatment: as for other types of RA.

Herbal options: Hormone stimulants and regulators will commonly be prescribed along with the same sort of regime recommended for RA. Useful hormonal herbs include agnus castus and black cohosh with evening primrose oil worth taking in supplements as this can ease both menopausal problems and joint inflammations. Regular cups of stinging nettle tea also appear to help in some cases.

Valerian or vervain can be useful for easing the emotional upsets associated with menopausal problems, while sage and mugwort used in teas or tinctures can ease hot flushes and night sweats which may be adding to the stress.

Additional dietary supplements to consider include vitamins B-complex, C and E, additional calcium, magnesium, selenium and zinc and fish oils.

Psoriaritic Arthritis
As with bowel-related joint disorders, psoriaritic arthritis is classified as a seronegative arthropathy. Around 1% of the UK population develops psoriasis and around 1% of this group has psoriaritic arthritis (around 550,000 sufferers); the condition is more common in women. Arthritis usually affects the fingers and toes while the associated skin scaling is common in the scalp or may cause pitting in the fingernails.

Orthodox treatment: Treatment for psoriasis can involve such local applications as coal tar, dithranol or ultra-violet light although in severe cases anti-metabolite drugs such as methotrexate may be used. Arthritis treatment is generally as for RA using NSAIDs or stronger drugs as appropriate.

Herbal options: Like rheumatic and arthritic disorders a herbal approach to skin problems such as psoriasis will generally focus on cleansing herbs such as red clover, sarsaparilla, burdock or figwort, as well as liver stimulants such as barberry and vervain. The problem also has a psychological dimension so soothing nervines or Bach flower remedies can be appropriate too.

Cleavers cream can be useful for clearing psoriaritic patches while evening primrose or starflower oil is also worth using topically and internally. Dilute rosemary or juniper oils can be used for any arthritic pain. Devil's claw, lignum vitae and black cohosh will help with the associated joint inflammation.

Systemic Lupus Erythematosis
Systemic Lupus Erythematosis (SLE) is a multisystem disorder which can include arthritis in many joints, although in the longer term it can be a more serious problem affecting kidney, brain and other internal organs. The cause of the disease is unknown but it usually affects young women and can sometimes then become a lifelong problem.

Onset is often acute with fever, polyarthritis and a distinctive 'butterfly rash' across the cheeks. In other cases it can be more gradual with poor appetite, general malaise and skin problems and it can take years to diagnose. Confirmation generally comes from blood and immunological tests but it is not always that easy to identify positively.

Five-year survival rates for SLE are more than 90% today and many sufferers continue into old age—although often on an increasingly potent cocktail of powerful drugs.

Orthodox treatment: SLE is a major health problem which can involve and damage many of the body's organs. The joint problems can often be mild and usually respond to NSAIDs. However the more severe form of the disease, where other organs are involved, is usually treated with corticosteroids, often up to 20mg of predni-sone and higher (up to 100mg) if there is kidney or cerebral involvement. Immunosuppressive drugs are also used in the long term and in high doses. These drugs have significant side effects adding to the sufferer's problems.

Herbal options: Remedies vary depending on the individual and her predominant problems but is always holistic, seeking to strengthen the body, ease stress-related factors, and consider any emotional dimension rather than simply alleviating symptoms.

Anti-inflammatories, cleansing herbs and blood tonics are all likely to be used. These can be similar to the remedies used for RA but might also focus on circulatory system herbs like ginkgo and lime flowers. There might also be anti-viral remedies if recurrent infections and general weakness were a problem and tonifying remedies like gotu kola, aloe vera and ginseng. SLE is not an illness for home treatment but always needs professional help.

Long-term sufferers often seek alternative treatment as a means of reducing high doses of damaging steroids, in which case, herbs like borage, which help to strengthen the adrenal cortex, can be appropriate.

Rheumatism

Rheumatism is a very non-precise term used to describe the various aches and pains suffered in muscles. The label can include fibrositis which is an inflammation of fibrous tissue, especially muscle sheaths, which often affects the back muscles. It leads to pain and stiffness and is usually treated with NSAIDs. Muscle pain may also be referred to as 'myalgia', which just means pain in the muscles.

Orthodox treatment: Orthodox medicine will generally prescribe painkillers and NSAIDs along with topical warming rubs (widely available as non-prescription over-the-counter products).

Herbal options: The herbal approach usually involves the use of cleansing herbs to remove any chemical toxins lingering in the tissues as with forms of arthritis. Myalgia is also often treated with the same sort of gentle restorative nervines and analgesics which would also be used for neuralgia (nerve pain)—typically St John's wort, chamomile or valerian.

Diuretics, digestive stimulants, circulatory stimulants and laxatives are all likely to be found in Western herbal remedies for rheumatism. Herbal painkillers and anti-inflammatories may also be included and a typical prescription might include bladderwrack, black cohosh, bogbean or white willow.

External warming remedies, such as rosemary, black pepper, peppermint, thyme, horseradish or wintergreen oils, can be used to stimulate the circulation by encouraging blood flow to a particular area. In China, plasters soaked in stimulating oils like eucalyptus or camphor are popular over-the-counter products widely available for muscle pains and 'rheumatism'.

Backache
In this country backache is reckoned to be one of the most common causes of absence from work, visiting the GP or seeking alternative medical treatment. Certainly the number of over-the-counter remedies for backache is impressive.

Orthodox treatment usually takes the form of bed rest and painkillers but thorough investigation is also needed to identify the cause of the problem. These can range from pulled muscles and damaged discs (the spongy plugs that separate the vertebrae and act as shock absorbers), to poor posture, kidney disease, gynaecological problems or simply sitting in an awkward position for long periods.

Some sorts of backache are dignified by rather grander names: lumbago simply means pain in the lower back (the lumbar region) from whatever cause, whereas 'sciatica' is often applied to odd aches and pains in the back but is technically a pain felt along the back and outer side of the thigh, leg and foot, with accompanying back pain and stiffness, generally caused by a damaged disc putting pressure on either the sciatic nerve or one of the many other nerves which start in the lower back area. Both can cause severe pain and leave sufferers unable to straighten up. In acute cases immediate professional medical attention is often needed.

Obviously all these different sorts of backache require very different treatments so accurate diagnosis is important if therapy is to be at all relevant.

Muscular aches and stiffness can often be associated with recent strenuous exercise—gardening or DIY—or perhaps a period of overwork with too long spent bending over computer keyboards or desks. Similarly if the cause is associated with kidney weakness or a displaced uterus then these underlying problems need to be tackled first, as simple backache remedies will only ever provide symptomatic relief.

Orthodox treatment: Initially bed rest and painkillers are the usual choice followed by further clinical investigation and possibly surgery as appropriate.

Herbal options: Symptomatic relief using massage oils can often be very effective in minor, self-limiting problems associated with muscle strain and over-exertion. Rubs containing lavender, thyme, marjoram, and/or rosemary oils are ideal (see Chapter 5). Internally devil's claw is helpful for longer-term problems or white willow and black cohosh in more acute conditions.

For backache associated with kidney problems typical herbal remedies will include kidney tonics and diuretics, such as cinnamon or buchu, while uterine-related disorders might be treated with black haw bark or black cohosh.

If the problem is really originating from damage within the back itself then often treatment from an osteopath, chiropractor or acupuncturist can solve the problem. Massage from a remedial masseur or physiotherapist can also give relief while poor posture can be helped by learning the Alexander Technique through a series of lessons. Always bend at the knees rather than the waist when stooping to pick up something from the ground.

For persistent backache with no obvious cause changing sleeping arrangements can sometimes help. Firm mattresses can be worth trying, while alternatively lying on your back with knees bent or curling into a small ball with the spine curved as in the foetal position as you fall off to sleep can often bring relief. Putting an extra pillow under the mattresses to raise the top of the bed is also worth trying as is experimenting with the various orthopaedic pillows on the market.

Repetitive Strain Injury

The high-tech world of the 21st century is a major cause of upper back and shoulder pains with 'repetitive strain injury' (RSI) blamed for a variety of problems.

RSI has become a *cause célèbre* in recent years with organisations like the National Union of Journalists vociferously campaigning on behalf of members who, it is claimed, are suffering a lifetime of ill-health as a result of using computer keyboards for many hours each day. This sort of injury was first recorded among copper beaters in Ancient Babylon and over the centuries similar ailments such as 'upholsterer's hands' and 'fisherwoman's fingers' have regularly been categorised by occupation.

Any excessively repetitive task, be it typing, scanning bar codes in a supermarket, or playing a musical instrument can lead to physical problems. Taking regular breaks from work is often easier said than done but it is important to try and vary the routines which have contributed to the problem. By law anyone who has to spend lengthy periods at a computer keyboard must take regular breaks and ensure that chair heights are correctly adjusted, and that there is space between the keyboard and the desk edge to rest the wrists can also prevent long-term damage.

Repetitive strain injury often manifests as agonising cramp-like pain when attempting the slightest physical task. There may lso be a burning sensation in the hands, arms, shoulders or back leading ultimately to fatigue, an inability to work effectively and depression. Onset can be sudden with sufferers simply waking one morning to discover themselves virtually crippled.

Orthodox treatment: As with other disorders that can be hard to classify, many RSI sufferers have found it difficult to obtain appropriate treatment. Anti-depressants and tranquillisers are often prescribed with the sufferer dismissed as work-shy. More practical options can be NSAIDs and possible localised corticosteroid treatment but long-term relief can be elusive.

Herbal options: Appropriate herbal medicines will generally include anti-inflammatories and cleansing remedies, as with arthritic problems, but there will also be emphasis on tonic and immune-stimulating herbs, and relaxing nervines, such as vervain and valerian. Muscle-relaxing remedies generally used for muscle cramp, such as wild yam or lobelia, can also be worth trying. Suitable immune tonics include astragalus (*Huang Qi*), reishi or shiitake mushrooms and ginseng.

Baoding balls—Chinese massage balls slightly larger than golf balls—can help. These need to be rotated in the palm for 5–10 minutes each day, a slightly cumbersome skill that is not difficult to learn. This helps to massage the ends of many major acupuncture meridians and so can help to re-energise many of the body's organs.

Massage oils containing lavender, thyme, rosemary or eucalyptus can also provide some relief.

Soft Tissue Disorders

Problems such as tendinitis, tenosynovitis and bursitis are among the rheumatic diseases affecting soft tissue: the tendons, tendon sheaths, bursae, nerves and fat. Such disorders are very common and include an assortment of highly specific ailments such as housemaid's knee or tennis elbow.

Local tendinitis is often associated with excess exercise of that particular joint, typically the Achilles tendon (at the back of the heel), the rotator cuff region of the shoulder, the fingers, and the wrist—washerwoman's wrist was commonplace in the days when clothes needed to be wrung manually rather than laundered in an automatic washing machine.

Bursae are small sacs of fibrous tissue lined with synovial membrane and filled with fluid which help to reduce the friction in a joint. They are found wherever parts move over one another and are normally formed around joints and places where ligaments and tendons pass over bones.

Bursitis is generally associated with mechanical stress and damage and can also be an occupational hazard; housemaid's knee is bursitis in the prepatellar region of the knee, while ill-fitting shoes can lead to inflammation of the retrocalcanean bursa between the calcaneus and Achilles tendon at the back of the heel. Tennis elbow involves the radiohumeral bursa and is associated with the backward stretching of tendons—it is similarly known as miner's, golfer's, jogger's, tailor's or pudding-mixer's elbow.

Orthodox treatment: Rest and local corticosteroid injection are the usual orthodox treatments.

Herbal options: Externally massage with a mixture of 5ml of St John's wort oil containing 20 drops of chamomile oil and 10 drops of lemon oil can help to relieve local pain, discomfort and inflammation. Arnica creams and compresses soaked in dilute arnica tincture can also help. Internally a mixture of meadowsweet, lignum vitae, black cohosh and St John's wort can be taken along with devil's claw tablets and magnesium supplements. Acupuncture can help to ease pain in chronic or persistent cases and sufferers need to try to reassess their regular movements if possible to avoid repetition.

Traumatic Injuries
Traumatic injuries need immediate first aid as well as calming sedative remedies to help combat shock and anxiety. If they are the result of some accidental, traumatic injury then an X-ray may be necessary to identify fractures. Strains involve a slight tearing of a muscle or the tendon attaching it to a bone and are generally caused by over-stretching. Sprains are a tear in the joint capsule or associated ligaments caused by twisting.

Orthodox treatment: Little beyond rest and painkillers is generally recommended with support from elastic or tubular bandages often employed to help immobilise the joint.

Herbal options: Treatment for traumatic injuries generally

involves analgesic and anti-inflammatory herbs applied in ointments or poultices. Alternating heat and cold can help to bring out
bruises and encourage healing: typically the injured joint needs to
be soaked for three to four minutes in hot water containing heating
herbs like black pepper, rosemary or camphor, followed by immer-
sion in a basin of iced water, repeated for as long as the sufferer
can bear.

Although crude herbs are nowhere near as strong as patent
analgesics for easing pain, they can be effective in other ways to
promote healing and cell growth. Comfrey, for example, contains
a chemical called allantoin which has been shown to stimulate
and speed cell repair—hence the plant's old country name of
'knitbone'. Arnica increases the absorption rate from internal
bleeding so also stimulates repair, especially in bruises which are
caused by blood escaping from damaged underlying blood vessels
following injury.

CHAPTER 3

The Eastern Approach

While modern medicine sees arthritic disorders largely in terms of inflammation and Western herbal medicine generally emphasises the need for improving elimination and circulation, other cultural traditions take a quite different view.

Chinese Traditional Medicine
In Chinese theory the various components of the musculo-skeletal system are each associated with specific elements and particular organs in a complex pattern that originated around 5,000 years ago. Traditional Chinese medicine is based on ancient Taoist principles which date back to the legendary emperor Fu Xi, believed to have lived around 3,000 BC. Fu Xi gave the Chinese a universal philosophy to interpret and explain all natural phenomenon. He was followed by Shen Nong—the divine farmer—who first taught mankind how to cultivate grains and is reputed to have personally tasted hundreds of herbs to identify their healing properties. Completing this legendary triumvirate was Huang Di, the Yellow Emperor, the supreme ruler of the universe, who introduced music, medicine, mathematics, writing and weapons.

Just as the ancient Greeks believed that all things were composed of earth, air, water and fire, so the Chinese applied similar logic and decided that all matter was made up of earth, metal, water, wood and fire. These elements were seen as closely interrelated, influencing and controlling each other, and were also matched to a lengthy series of other phenomena all grouped in fives: five solid body organs, five emotions, five seasons and so on (see Table 2). In Chinese theory it is important to maintain balance between the five elements as excess or weakness of any of them can affect the

Table 2: Five-element associations

	Wood	Fire	Earth	Metal	Water
Direction:	East	South	Centre	West	North
Colour:	Green	Red	Yellow	White	Black
Season:	Spring	Summer	Late Summer	Autumn	Winter
Climate:	Wind	Hot	Dampness	Dryness	Cold
Solid organ:	Liver	Heart	Spleen	Lung	Kidney
Hollow organ:	Gall Bladder	Small Intestine	Stomach	Large Intestine	Urinary Bladder
Sense organs/ openings:	Eyes Sight	Tongue Speech	Mouth Taste	Nose Smell	Ears Hearing
Emotion:	Anger	Joy/ Fright	Worry	Sadness/ Grief	Fear
Taste:	Sour	Bitter	Sweet	Pungent/ Acrid	Salty
Tissues:	Tendon	Blood vessels	Muscles	Skin	Bone
	Nails	Complexion	Lips	Body hair	Head hair
Sound:	Shouting	Laughing	Singing	Weeping	Groaning
Smell:	Rancid	Burnt	Fragrant	Rotten	Putrid
Body fluid	Tears	Sweat	Saliva	Mucus	Urine
Meat	Chicken	Mutton	Beef	Horse	Pork
Cereal	Wheat	Glutinous millet	Millet	Rice	Beans

balance of any of the associated factors; this in turn could upset the inner harmony both of the universal and individual beings.

As well as this five-element model, early Chinese physicians also saw well-being and illness in terms of *yin* and *yang*—two basic creative forces central to all things. *Yin* and *yang* have been compared to the light and dark sides of the mountain, the above and below, or the outside and inside; essentially they are paired and inseparable opposites vital to all things and contained within all things.

Elemental Influences on Muscles and Bones

In this five-element model, muscles are linked with earth and the spleen, bones with water and the kidneys, and tendons with wood and liver. Disorders in these tissues are therefore taken to imply some underlying weakness or imbalance in the associated solid (*Zang*) and hollow (*Fu*) organs.

In traditional Chinese medicine (TCM) these organs often have quite different properties from the conventional Western anatomical view. The liver, for example, is believed to 'store blood' while the spleen plays an important role in digestion separating the clear fluids (to be recycled) from the 'turbid' fluids which are excreted.

As with traditional Western theories, muscle pains are thus linked to poor digestion and a failure of the spleen to clear unwanted 'turbid' fluids (*Ye*). The connection between tendons and the liver is often apparent in chronic knee disorder: the knee has more tendons than other parts of the body and aching knees in the morning after an evening of excess alcohol and rich foods—putting extra strain on the liver—are very common.

Joint and muscle pains can thus be caused by internal imbalance and weakness and would be treated not with anti-inflammatories but with herbs to strengthen the relevant *Zang-Fu* organs. The kidney, for example, is associated with reproduction and creativity and its inner vital energies run down as we reach old age. Attributes linked with kidneys (such as head hair and hearing) decay as well and, since the kidney is associated with bones, osteoarthritis or osteoporosis are thus to be expected. All these old-age-associated problems would be treated with kidney tonics: these include commonplace herbs like cinnamon and walnuts as well as more exotic products like caterpillar fungus (*Cordyceps sinensis*). Problems with knees and tendons might be treated with liver herbs like *Dang Gui* (Chinese angelica), *Bai Shao Yao* (white peony) or *Huai Niu Xi*. Persistent rheumatism is likely to be associated with deficiency in spleen energy and problems it thus has in separating the *Jin* (clear) and *Ye* (turbid) products of digestion, so this would be treated with spleen tonics such as *Bai Zu*.

As well as these internal factors and imbalances, muscular aches and pains are also attributed to attack by external evils, rather like common colds. Wind is one of the main culprits and traditional Chinese theory sees a shifting pattern of twinges and aches and pains as typical of the variable nature of wind. Cold and damp are also common causes. Again this is something even sophisticated 21st-century Westerners can appreciate with arthritic and rheumatic pains often worse when the weather is wet or particularly cold.

Many of the herbs used for aches and pains—such as *Du Huo* (a type of angelica) and *Gui Zhi* (cinnamon twigs)—are the same as those used for common colds associated with external evils.

In Chinese theory arthritis can also be seen as attack by a combination of external evils: osteoarthritis, for example, is usually a cold–damp–wind problem with a shifting pattern of aches and twinges; symptoms are usually worse when the weather is cold and wet and the natural bone weakness likely in old age (due to the run-down in kidney energy) makes elderly people more susceptible.

Bi Syndrome and Arthritis

In Chinese theory if these external pathogens (such as cold or damp) move inside the body, they can cause obstructions in the acupuncture meridians, which run through the body, leading to pain and distension. If the limb meridians are afflicted then *Bi Zheng* is the result: *Bi* is usually translated in the West as 'pain' and *Bi Zheng* as 'painful obstructions'. Although the term can refer to any disease associated with obstruction, *Bi Zheng* is usually taken to mean diseases which in the West would be classified as arthritis or rheumatic disorders.

TCM suggests four prime causes for *Bi Zheng*, with different external pathogens affecting the meridians:

- wind obstructions, where the shifting nature of wind is the key differentiator and the pain moves from joint to joint; there may also be fevers and chills;
- cold obstructions, where the characteristics of cold predominate—fixed, stiff with severe pain that is worse in cold weather and on movement; the pain is relieved by a hot compress;
- damp obstructions, where the pain is usually fixed and there is swelling and numbness in the affected joints, joints feel heavy and numb and the pain is worse in damp weather; and

- hot obstructions, where the condition is characterised by joint swelling, pain and feverishness.

These basic forms of *Bi Zheng* usually exist in combination so that the sort of osteoarthritis or rheumatic pains of old age are generally some combination of wind–cold–damp while rheumatoid arthritis is usually a hot form—sometimes in heat–damp or wind–heat combinations.

With a variety of different 'evils' involved, herbs to treat painful obstructions can include cooling, drying and warming remedies with the combination selected to match the specific syndrome, age and constitution of the patient and stage of the illness. Many of the herbs used for arthritic problems are tonics for the liver or kidney used to strengthen their associated tissues from the five-element model. For the muscular aches and pains of rheumatism, spleen tonics would be used instead since the spleen is associated with muscles.

Herbs in this group would usually be described in the West as anti-inflammatory or analgesic. *Qin Jiao*, for example, has been shown in laboratory trials to be a significant anti-inflammatory, while *Cang Er Zi* was found in one trial involving lower back pain sufferers to ease pain in almost 90% of cases.

Tiger bones (*Hu Gu*), one of the more unsavoury forms of Chinese medicine, rightly condemned in the West for the threat it poses to the survival of tigers in the wild, are traditionally used for painful joint conditions. They are now known to be highly anti-inflammatory and to combat experimentally induced arthritis in laboratory animals, which accounts for their persistent use and popularity in many parts of Asia despite Western pressure to end the illegal tiger trade.

It is important to differentiate between the variants of *Bi Zheng* to find an appropriate remedy. The wind–cold–damp variety, for example, might be treated with a medicine like *Gui Zhi Shao Yao Zhi Mu Tang* (*Tang* simply means soup or decoction). This uses warm, drying herbs like cinnamon twigs (*Gui Zhi*) and ginger modified with a type of lily, *Zhi Mu* (a cold, bitter remedy) to keep the balance; liver and kidney tonics like *Bai Shao Yao* (white peony) are included to help strengthen tendons and bones. The remedy takes its name from its principle three herbs (literally cinnamon–peony–lily soup).

This would, however, be totally inappropriate for an arthritic problem associated with hot, inflamed joints, feverishness or associated skin rashes that would be attributed to a hot obstruction in the meridians. This hot form of *Bi Zheng* can be identified with rheumatoid arthritis although other less severe types of joint pains can also be attributed to hot conditions:

- wind–heat *Bi* syndrome is characterised by sore joints, stiffness and difficult moving, with a fever and thirst. The tongue is a darkish red with a yellow coating and the pulse will be rapid.
- damp–heat *Bi* syndrome also has fever and thirst, but skin eruptions are more likely and the joints will be more swollen and painful.

In rheumatoid arthritis there is often a changing pattern of symptoms and either of these varieties could be more dominant from time to time with wind–heat–damp *Bi Zheng* likely to show a variable combination of these symptoms.

One of the main remedies for damp–heat forms of *Bi Zheng* is *Er Miao San*, or 'powder of two effective ingredients', which is made up of *Huang Bai* and *Cang Zhu*. It is especially popular for pains in the lower back and knees linked to weakened liver energies. *Huai Niu Xi* can be included as additional support for the liver and knees and the mix is then known as *San Miao San* (powder of three effective ingredients). If dampness is a major problem, then *Yi Yi Ren* is added to the mix to create *Si Miao San* (powder of four effective ingredients).

Another popular remedy is *Bai Hu Jia Gui Zhi Tang* the 'white tiger decoction with cinnamon' which fortunately does not contain tiger bones. It contains cinnamon twigs (*Gui Zhi*), liquorice, and *Zhi Mu* along with gypsum and rice, and is used for treating arthritic pains associated with wind, heat and dampness where the symptoms include painful swollen joints which feel as though they are burning and are relieved by cold compresses or ice packs.

Shi Gao (gypsum or calcium sulphate) is one of the main minerals used in TCM. It is very cold and is used to clear heat in interior syndromes such as stomach fire problems and asthmatic conditions as well as heat obstructing the meridians.

Rice (*Oryza sativa*) is, of course, China's staple food. Rice seed (*Jing Mi*), sprouted rice (*Gu Ya*), and rhizomes (*Nuo Dao Gen Xu*) are used in medicine. *Jing Mi* is an energy tonic for spleen and stomach, *Gu Ya* is mainly for food stagnation, while *Nuo Dao Gen Xu* is for feverish conditions linked to kidney weakness.

Ayurvedic Approaches to Treatment
Ayurvedic medicine has its roots in the original Dravidian culture of India (c.5,000 BC), while the earliest surviving literature—the *Rig Veda* dating from around 2,500 BC—includes information on surgery, the use of prostheses and lists 67 medicinal herbs.

The basic medical theories of Ayurveda were extended and codified during the 1st to 2nd centuries AD with the middle ages bringing new medicines in the form of minerals and metal-based drugs. By the 16th century Moghul and European invaders had reintroduced Western ideas (in the form initially of Greek Galenic medicine known to the Moslems as *Tibb* or *Unani*) and Ayurveda went into decline. Pressure for Indian independence in the 1920s brought a revival of many traditional practices and today Ayurvedic medicine is taught alongside Western theory in many Indian universities. There are currently believed to be around 250,000 Ayurvedic practitioners in India ranging from university-trained medics to traditional healers.

Like the traditional medicine practised in the West from ancient Greek times until the 17th century, Ayurvedic health care centres on creating balance between bodily fluids known as humours. In Ayurveda there are three (*tri doshas*): *pitta* (bile linked to the fire element), *vata* (wind associated with the air and aether elements) and *kapha* (phlegm or dampness, ruled by the elements of water and earth).

Also vital is *prana*—the inner life force—which Ayurvedic practitioners feel at a pulse. The life force gives rise to fire: the fire of digestion and mental energy and *prana* is also linked to breath or oxygen which feeds the fire. If the fire is weak, then the body is weak. This inner fire is called *agni* or *tejas*, while the relationship between *prana* and *tejas* gives rise to *ojas* or good digestion and thus health. This good digestion is equated with juice or sap and this sap in turn produces the six experiences or tastes that are crucial in Ayurvedic herbalism. The three humours can also be seen as the waste products of the digestion process—the end product of the *prana–tejas–ojas* interaction. The more imperfect the digestion, the more waste products (*ama*) there are and the more imbalances in the system.

As well as harmony among the *tri doshas*, healthy balance also requires the seven *dhatus* or tissues to be in equilibrium. These are: plasma (*rasa*), blood (*rakta*), muscle (*mamsa*), fat (*medas*), bone (*asthi*), marrow and nerve tissue (*majja*), and semen (*shukra*). There are also numerous *srotas* or 'channels' which must be open allowing breath, food and water to flow freely into and around the body. They include familiar organs like the oesophagus, trachaea, arteries, veins and intestines, but the *srotas* can also be compared with the Chinese acupuncture 'meridians' which allow energy to flow around the body. There are the three waste products or *malas*—urine, sweat and faeces—which need to be in balance. *Agni*, the spirit of light or life energy, more prosaically interpreted as digestive function, also needs to be strong. Food, drink, sensual gratification, light, fresh air and spiritual activities all 'feed' *agni*, helping to maintain the balance of the *tri doshas* and ensure correct function of *dhatus*, *malas* and *srotas*.

The seven *dhatus* or tissues are each linked to particular humours; most (skin, muscle, fat, marrow and semen) are associated with *kapha*, but blood (*rakta*) is a *pitta* tissue and bones (*asthi*) are associated with *vata*.

Humoral imbalance or particular humour-related disorders are therefore likely to affect the associated tissues so problems with muscles and bones are not regarded as local, isolated disorders but are interpreted in terms of general health imbalance and treated accordingly. However, any humour can affect any tissue so although particular tissue problems are more likely when particular humours are in excess—as with bone disorders in old age when *vata* dominates—they can also be affected by imbalances elsewhere. As in traditional Western medicine, Ayurveda also links muscle (*mamsa*) and bone disorders with toxins building up in the system because of poor *agni* (digestive fire). Treatment for rheumatism or arthritis will therefore always involve a suitable dietary regime to correct the humoural imbalance as well as herbs to stimulate *agni* and clear toxins. Muscles (*mamsa*) are associated with *kapha* (water) so muscle problems can be associated with *kapha* imbalance which is more likely in damp climates. It is treated with warm, drying herbs as well as low-*kapha* diets (avoiding excess sweet foods, refined carbohydrates etc.).

As with Chinese theory, muscular aches and pains can develop from both internal (usually excess *ama*—toxin) or external causes. External problems can similarly be linked to the weather and the *vata*-type arthritis of old age is usually more prevalent in windy, damp or stormy conditions. Arthritis is generally associated with toxic *vata* (*amavata*) since the bones (*asthi*) are most closely associated with this humour. As in the Western herbal approach it can be linked to sluggish digestion leading to a build-up in waste products. Treatment of osteoarthritis often involves a *pitta*-promoting diet with hot spices to encourage *agni* (digestive fire) and burn off the toxic *ama*. 'Hot' gemstones such as rubies or garnets set in gold are also worn.

Ayurveda sub-divides arthritis into *pitta*, *vata* and *kapha* types, with rheumatoid arthritis most similar to the *pitta* type. This is treated with cooling, bitter herbs—such as aloe vera—rather than *pitta*-promoting remedies recommended for osteoarthritis (*vata*- or *kapha*-types); sandalwood or *gotu kola* are used in medicated oils for external massage.

Medicated oils are also used in Ayurveda to loosen stiff joints and clear toxins. *Mahanarayan* oil, where the main ingredient is *shatavari*, is one of the more popular for improving joint flexibility and is used regularly by dancers and athletes. *Narayan* oil (based on *ashwagandha*) is also used for muscle and joint pains and is believed to improve circulation. A household alternative is simply to use sesame oil which is a popular first-aid remedy for aches and pains in many parts of India.

In Ayurvedic medicine combinations of herbs are generally used in preference to simples with many traditional medicated jellies, pastels and pills widely available. Indian pharmaceutical companies are also researching many of these to produce effective remedies for the orthodox medicines market. Herbs are often taken in *ghee* (clarified butter) or milk to increase their tonic effects and there is also extensive use of medicated oils which are believed to be especially effective for strengthening specific *dhatus* (*rasa*, *rakta* and *mamsa*) and *agni*.

CHAPTER 4

Herbal Remedies for Joint Pains

Many types of herbs can be used in arthritis treatments; anti-inflammatories, analgesics, diuretics, laxatives, diaphoretics, metabolic stimulants and so on. How these are combined will depend very much on the underlying causes of the joint pains and any associated conditions.

Sometimes herbs are used singly—as devil's claw tends to be— but more often they are used in combination so that their varying predominant actions can be blended together. Not all herbal anti-inflammatories are also analgesic, for example, so it can be necessary to add remedies such as white willow, meadowsweet or black cohosh to an otherwise potent anti-inflammatory mix in order to provide some pain relief.

Some herbalists will limit their mixtures to four or five herbs, others may add up to 20 in a single prescription. In traditional Chinese medicine, practitioners use classic formulae for particular syndromes. These preparations have often been unchanged for hundreds of years and all Chinese medical students have to learn many hundreds of recipes by heart before qualifying.

For home use it is best to keep combinations as simple as possible limiting mixtures to two or three well-chosen herbs. As combining a few grams of herbs for a day's dosages can be complicated, use around 25–30g of each chosen herb, shake the dried herbs together thoroughly and store in a clean, dry jar. It is then easy to measure out 25g of the combination to make the day's dose of infusion or decoction as required. The same applies to combinations of tinctures—mix up 100ml each time, which is usually enough for a week's doses.

It can also be useful to combine external and internal remedies. Rosemary oil, used topically, for example, can bring fast relief for arthritic pains while devil's claw taken internally may need four or six weeks to start controlling the problem.

This chapter is organised into four sections:

- basic instructions for making herbal remedies at home;
- a section giving suggestions and examples for combinations of herbs for use in different types of joint and muscle pain;
- a detailed A–Z index of the major herbs used for treating joint pains; and
- a final section giving very brief details of all other herbs which are mentioned elsewhere in this book.

Making Home Remedies
Over-the-counter herbal remedies are readily available often in pre-mixed and proven combinations. Alternatively one can buy dried herbs and tinctures of single herbs and then blend them together to make the desired medicine. This can be quite simple and also very satisfying.

Infusions
An infusion is simply a tea made by steeping the herb in freshly boiled water for 10 minutes. Traditionally 1oz (25g) of dried herb was used to 1pt (500ml) of boiled water, which is sufficient for three doses, and the method can be used for most leafy herbs and flowers. The herb needs to be put into a ceramic or glass teapot or jug (with lid) and it is important for the water to just go off the boil otherwise many aromatic plant constituents will be lost in the excessive steam. After infusing, strain through a sieve as with conventional tea leaves, and take a wine-glass dose three times a day. Sweeten with a little honey if required.

If using fresh herbs one needs three times as much to allow for the additional weight of water in fresh plant material, i.e. 75g (3oz) to 500ml (1pt) of water.

The infusion can be reheated before each dose; this is helpful if the tea is being used for a 'cold' condition, such as chills or arthritis, although in many cases it can be drunk cold as well.

It is best to only make enough infusion for one day's doses, although any surplus can be stored in a refrigerator for up to 48 hours.

Decoctions

A decoction is like a tea but made by simmering the plant material for 15–20 minutes and is ideal for tougher plant components like bark, roots and berries, where it can be more difficult to extract the active ingredients.

Traditionally one used 1oz (25g) of herb to 1.5pt (750ml) of cold water which should then be brought to the boil in a stainless steel, glass, ceramic or enamel saucepan (not aluminium) and allowed to simmer until the volume has been reduced by about a third.

The mixture is then treated as an infusion: strained through a sieve and taken in three single wine-glass doses during the day. As with infusions, the tea can be warmed through before each dose and sweetened with a little honey as required, and it is best to only make enough for one day's doses at a time, although any surplus can be stored in a refrigerator for up to 48 hours. In China decoctions are always used instead of infusions with as much as 100g (4oz) or more of dried herbs heated in 500–1,000ml (1–2pt) of water.

Decoctions can be reduced down to 100–250ml with further heating and then this concentrated mix can be used in drop dosages either neat or in water.

Combined infusions and decoctions

When using a number of herbs in a tea it is often necessary to use some as infusions and some as decoctions—for example, if one were making a tea of lignum vitae with meadowsweet leaves for a rheumatic problem. In these cases it is best to measure out the required 750ml of water and use this to simmer the required amount of roots (perhaps 10 or 15g). Once the volume has reduced by about a third, pour the still-simmering mixture over the dried herb, in a jug, and infuse for a further 10–15 minutes. The tea can then be used as for simple infusions or decoctions.

Tinctures
A tincture is an alcoholic extraction of the active ingredients in a herb made by soaking the dried or fresh plant material in a mixture of alcohol and water for two weeks and then straining the mix through a wine press or jelly bag.

Commercially produced tinctures are usually made from ethyl alcohol with the supply of duty-free alcohol strictly controlled in the UK by H.M. Customs and Excise. Commercially made tinctures can sometimes be extremely expensive since, in Britain, the customs officials regard the more pleasant-tasting tinctures— including those made from lavender and rosemary—as in the liqueur category and thus liable to duty. Although any alcohol can be used to make tinctures, not all alcohols are safe to drink, so great care needs to be taken with home production. Methyl alcohol is extremely poisonous and, although some herbalists have used isopropyl alcohol (rubbing alcohol) for tincture making this, too, can be very toxic. Glycerol, which has the benefit of being very low cost, can be used but the resulting tinctures are slightly slimy to the taste. For home use, probably the safest and most accessible source of alcohol is in the drinks cabinet—spirits and wines.

Most tinctures are made from a mixture containing 25% alcohol in water (i.e. 25ml of pure alcohol with 75ml of water). This is slightly weaker in strength than most proof spirits such as vodka, whisky, rum, gin etc., so a suitable mixture can easily be made by diluting over-the-counter drinks. Of the commonly available spirits, vodka is generally considered the most suitable as it has fewer flavourings or herbal ingredients. Using rum is a good way to disguise the less palatable herbs. For a 37.5% alcohol mixture simply add a further 500ml of water to a 1-litre bottle of vodka to make 1,500ml of a 25% alcohol/water mixture that can then be used for tincture making.

Standard tinctures are usually made in the weight:volume proportion 1:5 (i.e. 1,000g of herb to 5,000ml of alcohol/water mixture or 1lb of herb to 5pt of liquid). For domestic use mixing 200g of herbs with 1,000ml of liquid is usually a sufficient quantity to make at any one time. If using fresh herbs then you need three times as much to account for the water content of the herb (i.e. 600g of fresh herb to 1,000ml of liquid). Some herbs, mainly roots, barks or those which contain a lot of resins or essential oils, need to be extracted in 45–60% alcohol mixtures. This is more difficult to obtain for domestic use. Using 25% alcohol will give a slightly weaker product when compared with commercial tinctures, although if using home-grown herbs their very freshness will more than make up for any loss of potency.

To make a tincture simply put the required quantity of herbs into a large jar (ideally an old-fashioned glass screw-top sweet jar). Then cover with the alcohol/water mixture and store in a cool place for two weeks, shaking the jar vigorously every couple of days. Strain the mixture through a wine press or jelly bag and store the resulting liquid in clean, dark glass containers. The herbal residue is an ideal addition to the compost heap.

Tinctures will generally last for two years or more without deterioration—although Ayurvedic medicine actually argues that the tinctures increase in potency as they age.

Fluid extracts
More concentrated alcohol/water extracts are available commercially as 'fluid extracts'; these are far more complex to make at home. The herb to liquid ratio is 1:1 and they are generally made by macerating the herb in five times its weight of liquid (as for a tincture) for up to two weeks and then heating the mix in a percolator to reduce the volume to around a half. This liquid is collected and reserved. Fresh alcohol/water is then added to the mixture and the cycle of maceration and percolating repeated twice more. Eventually the various liquid extracts are combined.

Because the alcohol will have evaporated during the process, fluid extracts do not last as long as tinctures and often need to have extra alcohol added for long-term storage.

Fluid extracts are, by definition, five times stronger than the average 1:5 tincture so need only be used in very small quantities. If the dose of a tincture is 5ml then 1ml of a fluid extract will deliver the same amount of herb.

Professional herbalists often use fluid extracts when large amounts of a herb are needed: meadowsweet, for example, used for pain relief in rheumatic disorders, is often given in fluid extract form.

Some typical combinations

Although herbs can be taken as 'simples' (singly on their own rather than mixed with other herbs) most herbalists will use a combination to balance the remedy to the patient's needs. The combination might be simply anti-inflammatories or analgesics or there could be cleansing and digestive stimulants added if function is poor. Herbs like devil's claw and turmeric are often taken as simples although they may be used in combinations.

Backache and lumbago

Much depends on the cause of the problem: if there is kidney involvement then herbs like cinnamon and buchu can help. For an inflammatory problem then devil's claw and black cohosh can be more appropriate.

- Celery, buchu, bogbean, St John's wort and bladderwrack—combine equal amounts of tinctures and take 5ml, three times daily.
- Black cohosh (3), turmeric (1), *Huai Niu Xi* (1) and meadowsweet (5)—combine tinctures in the suggested ratio and take 5ml, three times daily.
- Devil's claw (500–1,000g per dose) in capsules.
- Juniper (3), black cohosh (3), lignum vitae (1)—combine tinctures in the suggested ratio and take 20 drops, three times daily.
- Buchu, St John's wort and skullcap—mix equal amounts of dried herb and use one teaspoon per cup for infusions; add a pinch of powdered cayenne or black pepper to each dose.

Fibrositis

Although this term can be used synonymously with muscular rheumatism it implies a greater degree of inflammation and commonly affects the neck and back.

- Devil's claw (500–1,000g per dose) in capsules.
- White willow (6), black cohosh (2), and St John's wort (2)—combine tinctures in the suggested ratio and take 5ml, three times daily.
- White willow (6), cramp bark (2), and lignum vitae (1)—combine tinctures in the suggested ratio and take 5ml, three times daily.
- Bladderwrack, black cohosh, rosemary, meadowsweet and St John's wort—combine equal amounts of tinctures and take 20 drops, three times daily.

Osteoarthritis

In most cases cleansing and digestive stimulant herbs are combined with anti-inflammatories and analgesics. In addition liniments and massage oils (see Chapter 5) can help to give symptomatic relief.

- Celery seed, St John's wort, bogbean, yellow dock, angelica and prickly ash—combine equal amounts of tinctures and take 5ml, three times daily.
- Yarrow, boneset, elder—combine equal amounts of dried herbs and use 1–2 teaspoons per cup of infusion to encourage sweating and elimination.
- Black cohosh, bladderwrack, bogbean, devil's claw —combine equal amounts of tinctures and take 5ml, three times daily. Add *Huai Niu Xi* to the mix if the problem relates to the knees, hips or lower back.
- Devil's claw (500–1,000g per dose) in capsules.

Rheumatism and myalgia

Symptoms can vary from vague muscular aches to severe pain that will respond to strong analgesics like yellow jasmine. Black cohosh and St John's wort can be used in many cases.

- Black cohosh, meadowsweet, angelica, and burdock—combine equal amounts of each and use in tea three times daily. Add a pinch of cayenne or cinnamon to each cup to stimulate the circulation if need be.
- Bogbean (4), white poplar (4), sarsaparilla (2), lignum vitae (1)—combine tinctures in the suggested ratio and take 5ml, three times daily.
- St John's wort, black cohosh, yellow dock, burdock—combine equal amounts of tinctures and take 5ml, three times daily.
- Black cohosh, white willow, wild yam, celery and bogbean—combine equal amounts of tinctures and take 5ml, three times daily.

Rheumatoid arthritis

Combinations are likely to vary significantly between patients depending on the stage of the disease and symptoms. Likely options include:

- Celery, yarrow, angelica, black cohosh, prickly ash, meadowsweet, bogbean, white willow—combine equal amounts of tincture and take 5ml, three times daily.
- Lignum vitae, cleavers, dandelion root and skullcap—reported (Beatty, 1999) by one practitioner as bringing rapid and dramatic improvement to a case of early-onset RA.
- Celery and lignum vitae are ideal as a tea: use one teaspoon of celery seed and half a teaspoon of lignum vitae chippings to 250ml of boiling water. Infuse for 20 minutes, strain and drink during the course of the day.
- Stinging nettle (5), turmeric (1), lignum vitae (1) —combine tincture in the suggested ratio and take 2.5ml/ 50 drops, three times daily.
- Devil's claw (500–1,000g per dose) in capsules.

Sciatic problems
Sciatica often responds to manipulative treatments such as osteo-
pathy or chiropractic to deal with any displacement of the discs
which can be causing pressure on the sciatic nerve. Herbal remedies cannot repair the mechanical damage but can be helpful
where neuritis (nerve inflammation) is involved.

- Black cohosh (4), prickly ash (1), yarrow (2) and
  St John's wort (2)—combine tincture in the suggested
  ratio and take 5ml, three times daily.
- Use equal amounts of prickly ash and black cohosh in
  decoctions—one teaspoon of the mix per cup three times
  daily.
- Celery, barberry, buchu and valerian—combine equal
  amounts of tinctures and take 5ml, three times daily.
- Bogbean, white willow, St John's wort and passion
  flower—combine equal amounts of tinctures and take 5ml,
  three times daily.

Tendon and bursa problems
External treatments are often most effective but anti-
inflammatories taken internally can also help.

- Devil's claw (500–1,000g per dose) in capsules.
- Cramp bark and valerian—use equal amounts in a
  decoction; one cup, three times daily.
- St John's wort, skullcap and white willow—combine
  equal amounts of tincture and take 5ml, three times daily.
- Black cohosh, meadowsweet, and valerian—combine
  equal amounts of tincture and take 5ml, three times daily.

A–Z Index of Key Herbs

Angelica
Botanical name: *Angelica* spp.
Parts used: leaves, root
Taste: mainly pungent
Character: warm, dry

Actions: *A. archangelica*—carminative, diuretic, anti-fungal, anti-bacterial, diaphoretic, expectorant, digestive stimulant, anti-spasmodic, digestive tonic, smooth muscle relaxant; *A. pubescens*—anti-rheumatic, analgesic, anti-inflammatory, sedative, hypotensive, nervous stimulant
Dosage: up to 5ml of tincture daily
Caution: avoid in hot conditions and in pregnancy

European angelica (*A. archangelica*) is a warming, stimulating herb used in many types of cold conditions to increase body heat. The herb can be added to remedies for osteoarthritis and rheumatism where the condition is worse in cold, damp weather.

Angelica is mainly used as a digestive and circulatory stimulant so can help improve elimination and clear toxins from the system. It is effective for indigestion and colic and is also a specific for Buerger's disease where there is narrowing of the arteries in the hands and feet.

Several other varieties of angelica are also used in herbal medicine: *A. polyphorma* var. *sinensis* is Chinese angelica or *Dang Gui* mainly used as a liver and gynaecological remedy and as a tonic in weakness and debility. *A. pubescens* (Pubescent angelica/*Du Huo*) is primarily used in Chinese medicine to combat attack by the external pathogens 'wind' and 'damp', so is helpful for superficial syndromes including colds and rheumatism as well as *Bi Zheng* (arthritis). It is especially used for 'wind–damp' problems affecting the lower half of the body, especially lower back and legs, which may manifest as cramping pains, dull aches or stiffness. It is also used for headaches and toothache associated with 'wind–damp'.

Asafoetida
Botanical name: *Ferula assa-foetida*
Parts used: oleo gum resin
Taste: pungent
Character: hot, dry
Actions: expectorant, carminative, anti-spasmodic, nervine stimulant, non-steroidal anti-inflammatory, anti-coagulant
Dosage: up to 10ml of tincture daily

Caution: do not use for young children or babies

Asafoetida, also known as devil's dung or *hingu* in Sanskrit, has been described as the most foul-smelling of all herbs, although others describe the resin as merely smelling of fresh truffles.

It is a potent digestive remedy, used in Ayurveda to clear food stagnation from the digestive tract and strengthen the digestive fire (*agni*). It is traditionally used as an anthelminthic to clear parasitic round worms and thread worms and relieves excess wind and abdominal bloating. The herb also helps cleanse the intestinal flora and is an ideal antidote to eating junk food. It is traditionally added as a spice to lentil and bean dishes to reduce the 'windy' nature of these foods and to stimulate the digestion, and is used as a flavouring in traditional Worcestershire sauce.

While asafoetida is largely used as a digestive remedy in traditional Indian medicine, it has also been used by Western herbalists to clear mucus and phlegm in bronchitis, asthma and whooping cough. It is calming and will reduce high blood pressure and relieve stress.

Externally, asafoetida paste is used in Ayurvedic medicine for arthritic joints and abdominal pain and its efficacy has been confirmed in clinical studies; in one 1966 study using the herb for a group of 30 patients suffering from either rheumatoid arthritis or osteoarthritis improvements were reported in 28 (quoted in Bartram, 1995).

Birch—see Chapter 5

Black cohosh
Botanical name: *Cimicifuga racemosa*
Parts used: rhizome
Taste: bitter, pungent
Character: cool, dry
Actions: anti-spasmodic, anti-arthritic, anti-inflammatory, anti-rheumatic, mild analgesic, relaxing nervine, sedative, relaxes blood vessels, promotes menstruation, diuretic, anti-tussive, reduces blood pressure, lowers blood sugar levels

Dosage: up to 2ml of tincture of 200mg in capsules daily
Caution: excess can cause nausea and vomiting and the herb should be avoided in pregnancy

Black cohosh is a traditional North American plant which arrived in Europe in the 19th century. It was very widely used by Native Americans for yellow fever, colic, 'hysterical affections', snake-bite, sore throats and kidney problems, as well as for an impressive list of gynaecological problems. Primarily, though, it was regarded as a remedy for rheumatism and as such it was a 'favourite remedy' of the 19th-century American eclectic physician John King (1813–93) who used it for both acute and chronic cases of rheumatism and for other inflammatory conditions including respiratory problems and neuralgia (Foster, 1999).

Studies during the 1950s and 60s identified its main constituents as various triterpene glycosides including xyloside and cimicifugoside as well as possibly isoflavone but much of this research has produced conflicting results and little is really known of its active principles.

As well as its use as a rheumatic remedy, more recent studies have focused on its gynaecological action and several (detailed in Foster, 1999) have confirmed that it effectively relieves menopausal symptoms. Researchers currently disagree as to its actual action with some suggesting that it has oestrogenic-like activity while others maintain it is non-hormonal. Whatever its action, the herb has been shown in trials to relieve all sorts of menopausal discomforts including hot flushes, sweating, sleep disturbances, emotional upsets and depression. As a result, it is rapidly becoming a popular over-the-counter remedy for menopausal problems, although it can also be helpful for breast discomfort associated with premenstrual syndrome. Traditionally the herb was used to prevent threatened miscarriage, although such use requires skill and experience and is not an area for home remedies.

Black cohosh is still popular for aches and pains and is included in many over-the-counter remedies for arthritis and rheumatism: it is also recommended for cramps, sciatica, back pain, facial neuralgia and aches and pains following strenuous exercise.

Black pepper—see Chapter 5

Bladderwrack
Botanical name: *Fucus vesiculosus*
Parts used: whole plant (thalli)
Taste: salty
Character: cold
Actions: metabolic stimulant, nutritive, thyroid tonic, anti-rheumatic, anti-inflammatory
Dosage: up to 1g in tablets or 20ml of tincture daily
Caution: bladderwrack will concentrate toxic waste metals such as cadmium and strontium which pollute our oceans and should not be collected in contaminated areas

Like many seaweeds, bladderwrack is a salty, tonic herb, rich in iodine and trace metals and a good source of essential nutrients. The iodine content stimulates the thyroid gland and thus speeds up body metabolism—hence seaweed's reputation as a slimming aid. Several seaweeds are marketed as 'kelp', including *Ascophyllum nodosum*, *Laminaria* spp. and *Macrocysris pyrfera*; like bladderwrack all are rich in iodine.

Stimulating the metabolism can help to burn off extra calories so bladderwrack is often promoted as assisting in weight loss. However, it is really only effective if a sluggish thyroid is part of the problem and excessive use can lead to thyrotoxicosis (overactive thyroid).

Bladderwrack is highly nutritious and a good source of sodium, manganese, sulphur, silicon, zinc and copper so it makes a good general metabolic tonic especially in debility. Studies also suggest it can reduce the risk of atherosclerosis by helping to maintain the elasticity of blood vessel walls. Bladderwrack can also combat the onset of osteoarthritis and rheumatism.

Externally infused bladderwrack oil (see Chapter 5) makes a very effective massage base for use in both rheumatism and arthritis.

Bogbean
Botanical name: *Menyanthes trifoliata*
Parts used: herb
Taste: bitter
Character: cold, moist
Actions: bitter, tonic, diuretic, anti-rheumatic, anti-inflammatory, lymphatic cleanser
Dosage: up to 15ml of tincture per day
Caution: avoid if suffering from diarrhoea or colitis; may cause vomiting in excess

Bogbean, an attractive, white-flowered water plant, is related to the gentian family and like that group of herbs is bitter and stimulating for the digestive system. It contains similar alkaloids to gentian, iridoid glycosides, flavonoids, and several organic acids, including salicylic acid (Swiatek *et al.*, 1986). Bogbean has long been used in folk tradition as a remedy for rheumatism and arthritis as well as to treat fluid retention and fevers. As a bitter, it was also once used as a substitute for hops in beer-making.

The herb is diuretic, laxative and stimulating for the digestion so makes an effective cleansing remedy for rheumatism and arthritis and combines well with celery, white willow or black cohosh. It is useful in gout, rheumatism and rheumatoid arthritis and is also tonifying so helps to combat any associated debility, weight loss or lack of vitality.

It can also be helpful for indigestion and anorexia but as a stimulating digestive remedy should be avoided by those suffering from chronic diarrhoea or irritable bowel syndrome.

Burdock
Botanical name: *Arctium lappa*
Parts used: leaves, root
Taste: bitter
Character: cool, dry
Actions: diuretic, depurative, laxative, lowers blood sugar, diaphoretic, bitter digestive tonic, anti-bacterial, anti-fungal
Dosage: up to 20ml of tincture daily

Caution: avoid in pregnancy and breast-feeding

Burdock is a common European plant familiar for its hooked burrs which get caught in clothing and animal fur. Both the root and leaves have long been used in the West as a cleansing herb for skin and rheumatic problems or where a sluggish digestion is contributing to a build-up of toxins. The herb also encourages sweating, helping to reduce body temperature and elimination. The seeds are traditionally used in China for treating feverish colds, although modern research also suggests some anti-microbial activity notably against staphylococcus infections. The plant has also shown anti-tumour activity in animal studies (Dombradi and Foldeak, 1966).

The root is regarded as rather more potent than the leaves and tends to be preferred for internal remedies for gout, rheumatic disorders and other arthritic problems, while the leaf is more often used both internally and externally for skin problems including psoriasis and acne.

The plant is often combined with yellow dock or dandelion to increase elimination with the three roots especially effective when used in decoctions (1 teaspoon of the mixture per cup) rather than as a tincture.

Camphor—see Chapter 5

Celery
Botanical name: *Apium graveolens*
Parts used: seeds, essential oil
Taste: bitter, sweet
Character: cool
Actions: anti-rheumatic, sedative, urinary antiseptic, anti-spasmodic, diuretic, carminative, lowers blood pressure, some anti-fungal activity reported
Dosage: up to 20ml of tincture daily
Caution: Celery seed contains bergapten which can increase the photosensitivity of the skin. The oil and large doses of seed should be avoided in pregnancy

Although it is the seeds of the celery plant that are mainly used as a medicinal herb, both stalk and root of this familiar vegetable do have some therapeutic properties: the root was once used to treat urinary stones, while the stalks are characterised in Eastern medicine as having a bitter-sweet taste making them a moist cooling food ideal to balance hot, drying, spicy chilli dishes.

The seeds will encourage excretion of uric acid, which is helpful for a number of arthritic conditions, especially gout. They also help lower blood pressure and are a reputed aphrodisiac.

The juice extracted from the whole plant and roots can be used as a tonic for debilitated conditions and may also help with joint or urinary tract inflammations (Gursche, 1993). The juiced stalks can also make a suitably cooling therapeutic drink in feverish conditions or during arthritic flare-ups; it blends well with carrot juice.

A volatile oil, extracted from the seeds, contains apiol which is a uterine stimulant, also found in parsley seeds, and for this reason large quantities are contraindicated in pregnancy. The stalks are, however, perfectly safe for expectant mothers and can also help stimulate milk flow after the birth.

Celery seed is found in a number of over-the-counter patent remedies for fluid retention and also in preparations for rheumatism and arthritis. The seed can be used in infusions, decoctions or ground in a peppermill and sprinkled over food.

Comfrey—see Chapter 5

Devil's claw
Botanical Name: Harpagophytum Procumberus
Parts used: tuber
Taste: bitter
Character: warm
Actions: anti-inflammatory, anti-rheumatic, analgesic, sedative, diuretic, digestive stimulant
Dosage: 750mg in capsules two to three times a day during acute periods reduced to 500g twice a day when the pain eases

Caution: devil's claw is believed to stimulate uterine contractions and should be avoided in pregnancy. It should also be avoided in cases of gastric or duodenal ulcer

Devil's claw is a native of the Kalahari desert in Southern Africa and has been used for centuries in Namibia for a wide range of ailments ranging from malaria and gallstones to childbirth and wounds. The herb reputedly came to the attention of Westerners in 1904 when a German farmer—Herr G. H. Mehnert—allegedly discovered its secrets from a medicine man during the Hottentot rebellion (Carle, 1990). The plant was sent to Germany for investigation and by 1958 its anti-inflammatory, analgesic and anti-rheumatic properties were well established. It is also a bitter remedy so helps to stimulate and tonify the digestion.

The herb takes its name from the long, barbed woody fruits which resemble a fistful of clawed fingers. The secondary storage roots and tubers are used medicinally and like many other newcomers to the Western herbal repertoire the plant tends to be used singly rather than in combination with other remedies.

The plant's main constituents are three iridoid glycosides called harpagoside, harpagide and procumbide as well as a group of phytosterols made up mainly of *beta*-sitosterol and stigmasterol. In addition the root contains various organic acids, essential fatty acids and flavonoids.

The herb is used for a wide variety of rheumatic complaints mainly arthritis and low back pain and it is also helpful for headaches and neuralgia. Several studies have shown that it can be effective for rheumatoid arthritis.

Studies have also suggested that in general short-term (less than two weeks) use of the herb has little effect and it needs to be taken for anything from six weeks to six months to bring about significant improvements in the movement of arthritic joints and reduction of any swelling (Belaiche, 1982; Lecomte and Costa, 1992). In some trials subcutaneous injections of an aqueous extract of the herb have been used and Belaiche (1982) used nebuliser sprays of the solution, although capsules containing the crushed root are more commonly used.

French work (Pinget and Lecomte, 1988) found significant reduction in pain in 89% of a group of 43 arthritis sufferers after taking devil's claw for 60 days. In 86% of cases there was also significant reduction in the time it took any joint stiffness to wear off. Side effects reported in this study were minimal with only two patients reporting nausea or abdominal bloating. Dosage in this study was 0.75g of devil's claw powder in capsules, twice a day.

Clinical trials have also demonstrated that devil's claw can be effective for low back pain: one trial at University Hospital in Heidelberg, (Chrubasik *et al.*, 1996) used two 400mg tablets of devil's claw extract, three times a day (equivalent to 6g of crude herb) for patients suffering from chronic back pain and seeking treatment for acute pain attacks. After four weeks, nine of the 51 patients taking devil's claw were totally free of pain compared with one in the control group taking a placebo.

Devil's claw can also be used as a bitter digestive stimulant for a range of liver and gall bladder disorders.

The herb is widely promoted as an arthritic remedy in health food shops but the products on offer are not always of the best quality. Only the secondary storage roots and tubers contain the active principles; poor-quality products may often be derived from the whole root structure so the resulting remedy is either less effective or even totally useless depending on the part of the plant used. Better-quality products will give details of harpagoside content and standardised products are available in Germany. External creams and lotions containing devil's claw are also promoted as remedies for joint pains although there is little research into their efficacy.

Interest in harpagoside and harpagide activity has also encouraged researchers to look for these chemicals in European herbs and it has been found in common figwort (*Scrophularia nodosa*) and in mullein leaves (*Verbascum thapsus*) (Weiss, 1988).

Feverfew
Botanical name: *Tanacetum parthenium*
Parts used: leaves
Taste: bitter

Character: warm, dry

Actions: anti-inflammatory, analgesic, anti-spasmodic, anthelminthic, cooling, digestive stimulant, emmenagogue, peripheral vasodilator, relaxant

Dosage: 1.5ml of tincture (in 20 drop doses) or 125mg in capsules, daily

Caution: not to be taken by those prescribed warfarin, heparin and similar drugs. Migraine sufferers should stop taking regular doses of feverfew if side effects (skin rashes or mouth ulceration) occur

Like comfrey, feverfew has hit the media headlines in recent years—this time as a major 'cure' and prophylactic for migraine and arthritis. Since the 1970s, the plant has been extensively researched and is known to contain parthenolides and sesquiterpene lactones which are believed to account for is action in easing the symptoms of both migraine and chronic arthritis. Pure parthenolide is known to inhibit the production of prostaglandins (Groenewegen *et al.*, 1992)—rather like many NSAIDs—while the sesquiterpene lactones are known to be anti-inflammatory.

As an anti-spasmodic it can be helpful for period pain and is useful for minor fevers.

Although there is some tradition of using feverfew for headaches this was largely in external applications; writing in 1640, the herbalist John Parkinson suggested that the leaves were too bitter and unpleasant to actually eat, so in order to treat headaches, he recommended that they should be made into a poultice and placed on the crown of the head. Today, rightly or wrongly, feverfew is one of the most popular over-the-counter herbs for treating migraines, although the bitter substances they contain do have a tendency to cause mouth ulcers in a significant number of users.

Clinical trials have well demonstrated its efficacy as a migraine remedy and many sufferers happily eat a couple of leaves a day as a prophylactic. The herb does, however, have anti-platelet activity reducing the blood's ability to clot so should not be taken by those on blood-thinning drugs.

Feverfew is also popular as an over-the-counter remedy for inflammatory forms of arthritis including well-advanced osteoarthritis where inflammation often follows the initial damage. However, given its side effect of mouth ulcers it is probably best avoided by those suffering from genetically linked forms of rheumatoid arthritis which can be associated with ulcerative colitis. (One patient of mine once reported that her husband—not a patient—had developed ulcerative colitis after using over-the-counter feverfew products for his migraines continuously for several months.) Research continues into its use as a remedy for rheumatoid arthritis although its popularity as an over-the-counter remedy suggests that many sufferers already find it helpful.

Huai Niu Xi
Botanical name: *Achyranthes bidentata*
Parts used: root
Taste: bitter, sour
Character: neutral
Actions: analgesic, diuretic, hypotensive
Dosage: 5–10g of crude herb in decoction
Caution: avoid in pregnancy and heavy menstrual bleeding

Huai Niu Xi translates as 'ox knees from the Huai River', which may be a description of its knobbled stems but also points to its use in Chinese medicine as a liver remedy. The liver is associated with tendons and, as there are a great many tendons in the knees, aching knees can often suggest stagnating liver problems.

It is used in traditional Chinese medicine (TCM) to invigorate blood circulation and clear stagnant blood, to strengthen sinews and bones by nourishing liver and kidney, and to ease various digestive problems including sickness and nausea (Yeung, 1985).

It is used in many traditional TCM prescriptions especially for pains in the back and lower limbs and can also be helpful added to arthritic remedies using Western herbs such as black cohosh and white willow, especially if these parts of the body are involved, as it appears to be a directional remedy helping to focus attention on the lower part of the body.

The European name of the plant is generally given as two-toothed amaranthus.

Lignum vitae
Botanical name: *Guaiacum officinalis*
Parts used: heartwood and gum resin
Taste: astringent
Character: cold
Actions: anti-rheumatic, anti-inflammatory, laxative, diaphoretic, diuretic, depurative, anti-psoriatic
Dosage: up to 10ml of tincture daily
Caution: subject to legal restrictions in some countries

Lignum vitae or guaiacum is generally sold as wood shavings or raspings and is extracted from the heartwood of a tree growing in the West Indies and Florida. The herb is primarily used for rheumatism, arthritis and gout and sometimes for upper respiratory tract infections.

In the early 16th century it was considered an effective remedy for syphilis. Oveido, an early chronicler of North American botany, recorded that 'Caribbean Indians cure themselves very easily' of syphilis using the plant, and as a result it became much in demand in Europe as venereal disease spread. While the growers and gatherers certainly profited, the plant was actually quite ineffective at treating any sort of venereal disease and it gradually fell out of use.

Lignum vitae is, however, very effective for all sorts of rheumatic disorders. It is especially helpful for inflammatory conditions, such as rheumatoid arthritis, and will reduce pain and swelling. As a diaphoretic it encourages sweating and elimination of toxins through the skin and it can also ease myalgia and gout. Some herbalists suggest that it can also help prevent further gout attacks (Hoffman, 1983) as well as combat the shrinkage of tendons in the hand that leads to Depuytrens contracture (Bartram, 1995).

Lignum vitae is a popular ingredient of many over-the-counter rheumatism remedies. One double-blind study lasting two months with 72 patients (Mills *et al.*, 1996) showed that pain was significantly reduced in those taking Rheumalex, an over-the-counter preparation made by Gerard House which contains willow bark, lignum vitae, black cohosh, sarsaparilla and poplar bark.

Lignum vitae tincture can also be used in external embrocations for rheumatic pain.

Meadowsweet
Botanical name: *Filipendula ulmaria*
Parts used: aerial parts, leaves
Taste: astringent
Character: cold, moist
Actions: anti-inflammatory, anti-rheumatic, soothing digestive remedy, diuretic, diaphoretic, antacid, astringent
Dosage: up to 5ml of fluid extract, three times daily
Caution: meadowsweet is best avoided by those sensitive to salicylates and aspirin

Meadowsweet's claim to fame is as the herb which gave us the name 'aspirin'. In the 1830s chemists first identified salicylic acid, extracted from willow bark, as an anti-inflammatory and analgesic and over the following years worked to produce a synthetic drug. By 1899, Bayer had finally patented the result and since salicylates extracted from meadowsweet had been involved in the development work, they named the drug aspirin after the old botanical name for meadowsweet—*Spiraea ulmaria*.

Crushed meadowsweet flowers certainly have an aspirin-like scent and it was used in Elizabethan times as a strewing herb to improve the smell of less than clean houses, as well as to flavour wine and ales. Meadowsweet has long been used in much the same way as the proprietary drug, for easing pains and feverish colds and as an anti-inflammatory for arthritic conditions. It is used for rheumatoid arthritis, osteoarthritis, gouty conditions, muscular rheumatism, lumbago and sciatica. Studies have suggested that as well as the anti-inflammatory action of its salicylates, meadowsweet also helps to improve the condition of connective tissues (Zeylstra, 1998).

Unlike aspirin, which can irritate the gastric lining and in pro-longed use lead to ulceration, meadowsweet is extremely soothing and calming for the digestive tract. It is ideal for gastritis, indigestion and heartburn and is sometimes even described as having anti-ulcer activity. Meadowsweet infusion is ideal for many minor stomach upsets and taken after meals is good to counter indigestion; for digestive problems it combines well with marsh-mallow and lemon balm.

Strong extracts of meadowsweet are used by professional herbalists in treating arthritis and rheumatism, although in mild cases a home-made infusion can be useful—increase the normal standard proportion up to 50g of dried herb to 500ml of boiling water. Meadowsweet is also useful in arthritis and gout to clear accumulated toxins and increase urination.

A recent audit of herbal practice (Beatty, 1999) suggested that meadowsweet tends to be combined most commonly with devil's claw, white willow, celery, bogbean or white bryony for arthritic problems.

Prickly ash
Botanical name: *Zanthoxylum* spp.
Parts used: bark, berries
Taste: pungent
Character: warm, dry
Actions: bitter digestive stimulant, anti-spasmodic, carminative, circulatory stimulant, anti-rheumatic, diaphoretic
Dosage: up to 5ml tincture three times a day
Caution: excess may interfere with anti-coagulant medication (e.g. warfarin and heparin) owing to high coumarin content in *Z. americanum*

Two species of prickly ash are used in Western herbal medicine in very similar ways although the active chemical constituents of the plants varies. *Z. americanum* comes from the northern US states while *Z. clava-herculis* is from more southern areas. Commercial supplies often make little differentiation between the species although the southern prickly ash tends to be more commonly used and has been more extensively studied. The northern tree contains coumarins while the southern has amides such as herculin and cinnamide (Newall *et al.*, 1996).

Prickly ash is a warming, spicy herb that can help to relieve pain and stimulate the digestion. It was known in much of North America as 'toothache tree' and was used by many native people as a remedy to relieve toothache and muscular aches as well as to reduce fevers.

Western herbalists use the plant primarily as a circulatory stimulant in disorders such as Raynaud's syndrome and intermittent claudication, as well as to improve the blood circulation where this is a contributory factor in skin or rheumatic disorders and combines well with bogbean and lignum vitae.

Rosemary—see Chapter 5

Sarsaparilla
Botanical name: *Smilax officinalis*
Parts used: root and rhizome
Taste: sweet, pungent
Character: warm, moist
Actions: anti-rheumatic, anti-inflammatory, anti-pruritic, diaphoretic, diuretic, antiseptic, metabolic stimulant, immunostimulant, hormonal, blood tonic
Dosage: up to 20ml of tincture daily
Caution: none noted

A number of closely related *Smilax* spp. originating in Central and South America are used medicinally and they include *S. regelii* (Honduran sarsaparilla) and *S. febrifuga* (Ecuadorian sarsaparilla) as well as the Mexican variety (*S. officinalis*).

The herb is regarded as an aphrodisiac and virility tonic in many parts of South America and contains a testosterone-like compound so can certainly boost male hormones. It also contains cortin, a hormone which regulates metabolism, and the herb is popular for improving athletic performance and combating impotence.

In Western herbal tradition, the plant is largely used as a cleansing remedy, anti-inflammatory and antiseptic that can be helpful for irritant and chronic skin problems including psoriasis. It can also be useful for rheumatism, rheumatoid arthritis and gout and it is included in several over-the-counter products used for arthritic problems.

The Chinese use similar species (*Smilax glabra, Tu Fu Ling*) for treating venereal disease and rheumatoid arthritis.

Stinging nettle
Botanical name: *Urtica dioica*
Parts used: aerial parts, roots
Taste: astringent, slightly bitter
Character: cool, dry
Action: antiseptic, anti-rheumatic, astringent, blood tonic, diuretic, expectorant, galactagogue, hypotensive, lowers blood sugar levels, important source of minerals, clears uric acid
Dosage: up to 5ml of tincture three times daily
Caution: none noted

Stinging nettles were once used in a rather bizarre treatment known as urtication which involved beating paralysed limbs with stinging nettles in an attempt to stimulate sensations. The same remedy was also recommended for rheumatic pains, while the Romans reputedly planted the small annual continental nettle (*U. pilulifera*) along British roads because they believe the country was so cold they would need to beat their bodies with nettles to keep warm.

Rather unusually a group of researchers at Plymouth Postgraduate Medical School has recently studied the effect of nettle stings on joint pain (Randall *et al.*, 1999). Of the 18 patients who willingly stung themselves repeatedly with nettles, 17 were sure that the treatment had helped and several declared themselves cured.

Nettles sting because the hairs on their stems and leaves contain histamine which is a potent skin irritant. Thanks to its ability to 'rob the soil' and concentrate minerals and vitamins in its leaves it is a good nutrient and makes a useful 'spring tonic' as well as a good supplement in iron-deficient anaemia. Processing fresh young nettles in a juicer is a good way to take an energising tonic or they can be cooked in soups (see Chapter 6) to help clear out the stagnations of winter.

The herb is used throughout Europe as a remedy for rheumatic conditions and several studies have highlighted its anti-inflammatory and analgesic activity (ESCOP, 1997 and references therein). One clinical trial (Ramm and Hansen, 1995) showed improvements in 70% of a group of 1,252 patients suffering from degenerative rheumatic disorders after taking a daily dose of 1.5g of dried nettle extracts for three weeks.

Nettles can be used externally in washes or infused oils for irritant skin rashes and the same oil can be used as the base for a massage rub for rheumatism. Internally, nettle tea is a popular folk remedy for rheumatism and can help to relieve the acute painful stage of gout. In pregnancy, nettle tea makes a useful additional source of calcium and iron and it stimulates milk flow when breast-feeding. Nettle tea can be helpful internally for allergic skin rashes, especially those connected with salicylate sensitivity. The plant will also reduce blood sugar levels so is a useful addition to dietary control of late-onset diabetes.

More recent research has shown that stinging nettle can effec-tively enhance the action of the anti-inflammatory drugs (Ramm and Hansen, 1996). One trial in Germany covering 40 patients taking the drug diclofenac (Chrubasik *et al.*, 1997) demonstrated significant reduction in the necessary drug dose. Half the study group continued with their standard dose of 200mg of diclofenac while the others took 50mg of the NSAID and 50mg of stewed nettle leaf.

The results were impressive with the diclofenac and nettle com-bination proving just as effective as the higher doses of the drug. Previous studies had shown that doses of 75mg of diclofenac were totally ineffective at controlling arthritic pain but in combination with stinging nettle the drug appears more active.

Turmeric
Botanical name: *Curcuma longa*
Parts used: rhizome
Taste: bitter, astringent

Character: hot, dry

Actions: anti-inflammatory, anti-oxidant, cholagogue, hepatoprotective, anti-allergenic, immunostimulant, cancer preventative, anti-fungal, anti-microbial (specific for *Salmonella* spp.), reduces cholesterol levels, stimulates bile production

Dosage: 250–1,000mg daily

Caution: turmeric can cause skin rashes in sensitive individuals and may increase sensitivity to sunlight

Turmeric—known as *haridra* in Sanskrit, *haldi* in Hindi and *Jiang Huang* in China—is one of the more familiar Indian spices used for flavouring and colouring curries and sauces. Traditionally, it is used in Ayurveda as a digestive, circulatory and respiratory stimulant, cleansing for the *chakras* (energy centres) and purifying for the body. It also helps to thin the blood and lower cholesterol levels in cardiovascular disease.

In folk medicine it is used more prosaically for scabies, poor eyesight, to encourage milk flow in breast-feeding, and for rheumatic pains. The flowers are used in parts of India for sore throats and indigestion.

Traditionally turmeric was taken in India as a digestive stimulant and to combat infections as in gastro-enteritis and food poisoning. Externally it was used with honey for sprains, bruises and arthritic pains or taken as a milk decoction to cleanse and improve the skin.

In traditional Chinese medicine the herb is mainly used as a blood and energy stimulant and is also regarded as analgesic. It is used to treat chest and abdominal pain as well as frozen shoulder and menstrual problems.

Turmeric is now also being used as an anti-inflammatory for arthritic conditions. This actions was first reported in 1971 (Srimal *et al.*, 1971) and subsequent tests (Srimal and Dghawan, 1973) have shown curcumin, one of its key constituents, to be as potent as phenylbutazone and almost as effective as cortisone. A few clinical trials using turmeric extracts for arthritis have followed; one (Deodhar *et al.*, 1980) showed that the herbal extract produced a greater improvement than phenylbutazone without the usual side effects of NSAIDs. A recent double blind trial (Chopra *et al.*, 2000) used a combination of *ashwaghanda*, *gugulla*, ginger and turmeric with 182 patients suffering from RA. Over 16 weeks patients taking the Ayurvedic mixture found that there was a significant reduction in joint swelling using the mix, although other factors such as tenderness and pain seemed less affected.

Topical application of turmeric extracts are also strongly anti-inflammatory with a 'cortisone-like' action (Mehra *et al.*, 1984) so may be worth considering in conditions like tennis elbow and other localised joint inflammations.

In view of these results some herbalists (Bone, 1991) now recommend use of the herb for inflammatory arthritic conditions and traumatic injuries although it is generally necessary to combine the herb with more analgesic remedies, such as white willow or meadowsweet, to provide symptomatic pain relief. As with celery, using ground turmeric as a culinary spice can be a useful way of treating mild joint inflammations.

White bryony
Botanical name: *Bryonia dioica*
Parts used: root
Taste: bitter
Character: hot
Actions: diaphoretic, expectorant, emetic, cathartic, anti-tumour, topically rubefacient
Dosage: up to 10 drops of tincture, three times daily
Caution: avoid in pregnancy and breast-feeding; only use externally, internal use should be by qualified practitioners only

Bryony is a potent, highly toxic, bitter purgative used in small quantities by qualified practitioners for rheumatic and respiratory disorders. Externally it is used in many warming rubs for muscular aches and pains or rheumatism, while in homoeopathic dilution shows quite different properties and is used as a cold and catarrh remedy.

White bryony is also known as English mandrake since it has an enormous root stock which looks rather like mandrake

(*Mandragora officinarum*) and it was once used as a substitute for this potent narcotic. Bryony roots carved into human form were often used as shop signs by 18th-century herbalists.

The herb was once popular for coughs and pleurisy although as it is so toxic other less heroic remedies tend to be preferred today. It is used with black cohosh for muscular pain while some traditional herbalists (Bartram, 1995) suggest small frequent doses for the acute stages of many rheumatic disorders.

White willow
Botanical name: *Salix alba*
Parts used: bark
Taste: astringent, bitter
Character: cool, dry
Actions: anti-rheumatic, anti-inflammatory, anti-pyretic, anti-hidrotic, analgesic, antiseptic, astringent, bitter digestive tonic
Dosage: up to 25ml of tincture daily
Caution: avoid in aspirin salicylate allergy

In European tradition the silver-leaved willow was associated with the moon so was regarded as especially cooling for all sorts of inflammatory disorders. In 1838 early researchers isolated salicylic acid from the bark as the key active principle. Its name is derived from the botanical genus of the tree (*Salix*) and the chemical was eventually synthesised as acetyl salicylic acid or aspirin.

White willow is an effective herb for clearing heat, especially from the joints, throat, eyes and urinary tract, and is also good as a general treatment for headaches. The plant, like aspirin, is used for relieving pain and reducing fevers and is helpful for rheumatism, gout, arthritis, feverish chills and headaches.

It is especially useful for inflammatory forms of joint disease, including rheumatoid arthritis, ankylosing spondylitis and gout, and its analgesic action generally helps to ease painful muscles and joints. Herbalists generally use a fluid extract, which is rather more potent than a tincture, in doses up to 5ml.

Unlike aspirin, willow (as with meadowsweet) can also be soothing for the gastro-intestinal membranes and it can be used for diarrhoea and dysentery. White willow makes a suitable alternative to low doses of aspirin often prescribed for heart attack patients and can be combined with lime flower to help reduce the risk of atherosclerosis and clot formation.

It combines well with lignum vitae, black cohosh or celery for rheumatoid arthritis or with yarrow, stinging nettles, celery and devil's claw for more general arthritic conditions (Beatty, 1999).

A–Z of Other Herbs Mentioned in Remedies

Agnus castus (*Vitex agnus-castus*)—also known as chaste tree reputedly from its action as a male anaphrodisiac, used by medi-aeval monks to reduce libido and lascivious thoughts. Agnus castus acts on the pituitary gland to increase the production of female sex hormones which are involved in ovulation so is extremely useful for menstrual irregularities and menopausal problems.
Actions: pituitary stimulant and hormone regulator, reproductive tonic, increases milk production, female aphrodisiac, male anaphrodisiac
Caution: excess can create the sensation of formication—a feeling of ants crawling over the skin

Agrimony (*Agrimonia eupatoria*)—an astringent, bitter herb useful for diarrhoea or to stop bleeding. It has a long tradition as a wound herb and was the main ingredient of 'arquebusade water' a 15th-century remedy for battlefield gunshot wounds. Agrimony is also diuretic and contains silica (see Chapter 7) which makes it a good healing remedy. It can be helpful in cases of food intolerance to help to restore normal gut function.
Actions: astringent, diuretic, tissue healer, stops bleeding, stimulates bile flow, some anti-viral activity reported

Aloe vera (*Aloe vera*)—while 'bitter aloes' is a purgative extract made from various species of aloe, Aloe vera yields a mucilaginous gel which is largely used externally as a wound healer and to relieve burns and skin inflammations including eczema and thrush. The gel is also made into a variety of popular over-the-counter

remedies, promoted as tonics and restoratives. A tropical plant, it can be grown as a houseplant in temperate climates.
Actions: purgative, stimulates bile flow, wound healer, tonic, demulcent, anti-fungal, styptic, sedative, anthelmintic
Caution: avoid in pregnancy as it is strongly purgative; high doses of leaf extracts may cause vomiting

Arnica (*Arnica montana*)—encourages tissue repair after injury so is ideal after surgery or for sprains and bruises. Internally it acts as a circulatory stimulant but is extremely toxic and is generally used only in dilute homoeopathic doses.
Actions: anti-inflammatory, healing, circulatory stimulant
Caution: only take in homoeopathic doses internally. Do not use on open wounds; it may occasionally cause contact dermatitis

Ashwaghanda (*Withania somnifera*)—known as *ashwagandha* in Hindi, withania or winter cherry is an important Ayurvedic tonic believed to increase vitality and clear the mind. It is mainly used in the West as a tonic for the elderly and to combat debility resulting from over-work and chronic stress. In India it is also used as a tonic in pregnancy.
Actions: tonic, sedative, combats stress

Astragalus (*Huang Qi; Astragalus membranaceous*)—an important Chinese tonic herb used to strengthen the body's defences, *Huang Qi* is now being used in the West as an immune-stimulant in AIDS treatment and for recurrent infections. The Chinese prefer astragalus root to ginseng as a tonic for the under-40s.
Actions: immune stimulant, diuretic, tonic, vasodilator, antipyretic, anti-viral

Autumn crocus (*Colchicum autumnale*)—a specific remedy for easing the pain and inflammation of acute gout. It is a potent, toxic remedy restricted to use by professional practitioners only. The herb is usually combined with a diuretic remedy and does not increase the excretion of uric acid so celery also needs to be given.

Actions: anti-gout, emetic, cathartic, non-steroidal anti-inflammatory
Caution: not for lay use

Bai Shao Yao (*Paeonia lactiflora*)—or white peony, is used in traditional Chinese medicine mainly as a liver remedy for menstrual problems and digestive disorders.
Actions: anti-bacterial, anti-inflammatory, anti-spasmodic, diuretic, sedative, hypotensive, analgesic, anti-coagulant, immune stimulant, lowers blood cholesterol, peripheral vasodilator, hypoglycemic, stimulates tissue repair, improved microcirculation
Caution: avoid in diarrhoea and abdominal coldness

Bai Zhu (*Atractylodes macrocephala*)—one of the main energy tonics used in Chinese medicine especially for spleen or stomach weakness. The herb has been used in China since the Tang Dynasty (*c.*650 AD). More recently it has been promoted as a remedy to control appetite, of use in weight control regimes.
Actions: anti-bacterial, anti-coagulant, digestive stimulant, diuretic, hypoglycemic
Caution: avoid in *yin* deficiency characterised by extreme thirst

Barberry (*Berberis vulgaris*)—the bark is used mainly as a liver stimulant and spleen tonic for problems associated with sluggish liver and digestion including skin problems and rheumatic disorders associated with poor elimination.
Actions: liver stimulant, bile stimulant, antiseptic, blood cleanser, digestive tonic, anti-emetic, hypotensive, uterine stimulant, antimicrobial, febrifuge, anti-inflammatory
Caution: avoid in pregnancy and diarrhoea

Benzoin—see Chapter 5

Black haw (*Viburnum prunifolium*)—like its relative cramp bark, black haw is primarily a relaxant useful as an anti-spasmodic to relieve cramping pains and also to calm the nerves. It seems more specific for the uterus than cramp bark, however, and will rapidly

94

relieve period cramps. Herbalists also use the herb for threatened miscarriage and related disorders.

Actions: anti-spasmodic, sedative, astringent, uterine relaxant, diuretic, lowers blood pressure

Boneset (*Eupatorium perfoliatum*)—is so called from its traditional use in North America as a remedy for flu-type fevers with their associated aches and pains. The settlers soon adopted the herb as a cure-all and it reached Europe in the 19th century. It encourages sweating so is helpful in cleansing regimes.

Actions: immune stimulant, diaphoretic, relaxes blood vessels, laxative, stimulates bile flow

Borage (*Borago officinalis*)—better known commercially as ''star flower'', borage oil is used much as evening primrose oil as an important source of essential fatty acids. The herb is a potent adrenal stimulant and is used by professional herbalists as a tonic for patients recovering from lengthy courses of steroid treatment. Externally the juice can be used to sooth itching skin rashes and eczema.

Actions: Leaves—adrenal stumulant, stimulates milk flow, diuretic, febrifuge, anti-rheumatic, diaphoretic, expectorant; Seeds—source of *gamma*-linolenic acid and *cis*-linoleic acid.

Caution: aerial parts of the plant contain pyroolizidine alkaloids which may cause liver damage and use of the plant is restricted in some countries.

Buchu (*Agathosma betulina*)—originates from South Africa where it was traditionally used as an external dusting powder to protect the skin. It has a distinctive blackcurrant flavour and is a popular remedy for cystitis and fluid retention.

Parts used: leaves

Actions: diuretic, diaphoretic stimulant; tonic and warming for the kidneys

Cang Er Zi (*Xanthium strumarium*)—literally means 'deep green ear seeds' and it is one of the herbs used to clean wind–damp which in Chinese medicine is seen as a common cause of both nasal catarrh and *Bi Zheng* or arthritic pain. It was first listed by Sun Simiao around 620 CE.

Actions: anti-bacterial, anti-fungal, anti-rheumatic, anti-spasmodic, analgesic

Caution: not to be used for headache or arthritic pains associated with anaemia or blood deficiency. It contains a chemical called xanthostru-marin which may be toxic in high doses leading to convulsions

Cang Zhu (*Atractylodes lancea*)—used in TCM for clearing damp-ness, both for internal damp problems associated with the spleen and for external damp linked to *Bi Zheng*. The famous 16th-century herbalist Li Shi Zhen recommended fumigation with *Cang Zhu* during epidemics as an important preventative.

Actions: carminative, diaphoretic, increases excretion of sodium and potassium salts, although it is not diuretic

Caution: avoid in *Qi* or *yin* deficiency associated with interior heat

Caterpillar fungus (*Cordyceps sinensis*)—a parasitic fungus which grows on a type of caterpillar, the herb is known as *Dong Chong Xia Cao* in China. The traditional remedy contained the dead larva, although today the fungus is more often cultivated on a grain base. In ancient China *Dong Chong Xia Cao* was kept exclusively for use by the Emperor and his household and was cooked with roast duck to make therapeutic meals.

Actions: anti-cancer, anti-asthmatic, adrenal stimulant, anti-bacterial, sedative

Cayenne—see Chapter 5

Chamomile—see Chapter 5

Cinnamon (*Cinnamomum zeylanicum*)—a warming herb that can be helpful for all sorts of 'cold' conditions including chills and rheumatic pains. It has been used for centuries to treat nausea and vomiting and is also helpful for many digestive problems including

diarrhoea and gastro-enteritis. The Chinese use the twigs (*Gui Zhi*) of a related species (*C. cassia*) to encourage circulation to cold hands and feet, while the inner bark (*Rou Gui*) is seen as more centrally warming and is used to treat cold problems associated with low energy, such as debility, rheumatic problems and kidney weakness.
Actions: anti-spasmodic, antiseptic, carminative, warming digestive remedy, diaphoretic, tonic; essential oil—anti-bacterial and anti-fungal
Caution: avoid in pregnancy

Clary sage—see Chapter 5

Cleavers (*Galium aparine*)—usually dismissed as a weed, cleavers can be found scrambling through shrubs in most suburban gardens. It is an important lymphatic cleanser once used to feed domestic geese—hence its country name, 'goosegrass'.
Actions: diuretic, lymphatic cleanser, mild astringent

Cramp bark (*Viburnum opulus*)—a useful relaxant for both muscles and nerves. It can ease the spasms of cramp and colic and is also helpful for constipation. It can help with high blood pressure by relaxing blood vessels. Externally it can be used in creams and lotions to relieve muscle cramps.
Actions: anti-spasmodic, sedative, astringent, muscle relaxant, nervine

Cypress—see Chapter 5

Dandelion (*Taraxacum officinale*)—a comparative newcomer to Western herbalism, first mentioned in the 15th century. The plant is strongly diuretic so is often used for fluid retention and urinary problems. The root is also very cleansing for the liver and a mild laxative; it is often used in chronic skin problems and arthritis.
Actions: Leaves: diuretic, hepatic and digestive tonic; root: liver tonic, stimulates bile flow, diuretic, laxative, anti-rheumatic

Dang Gui—see **Angelica** page 71

Elder (*Sambucus nigra*)—once regarded as a complete medicine chest since all parts of the plant could be used in some way; today only the flowers are widely used, although berry juice is available. Elderflowers appear to strengthen the mucous membranes of the upper respiratory tract so, although some argue that the herb can cause hay fever, it can also increase resistance to irritant allergens.
Parts used: flowers, berries
Actions: Flowers: expectorant, anti-catarrhal, circulatory stimulant, diaphoretic, diuretic; locally: anti-inflammatory; berries: diaphoretic, diuretic, laxative

Eucalyptus—see Chapter 5

Evening primrose (*Oenethera biennis*)—a North American plant which was traditionally used in infusions for asthma and digestive disorders. During the 1970s researchers identified that its seeds were rich in *gamma*-linolenic acid (GLA), an essential fatty acid (see Chapter 8).
Actions: anti-eczema, demulcent, anti-thrombotic
Caution: do not take the oil if suffering from epilepsy

Fennel—see Chapter 5

Fenugreek (*Trigonella foenum-graecum*)—familiar from Indian and Middle Eastern cookery, and the herb gives a spicy flavour to curries, pickles and garnishes. The seeds are mainly used in herbal medicine as a warming remedy for stomach and kidney chills and it can be helpful in late-onset diabetes to reduce blood sugar levels. The whole dried plant is used as a tea in modern Egypt as a remedy for spasmodic abdominal pain due both to digestive upsets and menstruation.
Actions: anti-inflammatory, digestive tonic, stimulates milk production, locally demulcent, uterine stimulant, hypoglycaemic
Caution: avoid in pregnancy as it is a uterine stimulant. Insulin-independent diabetics should not take the plant without professional advice

Figwort (*Scrophularia nodosa*)—mainly used for skin eruptions and swollen glands. Figwort is helpful whenever toxins are contributing to the condition and is generally cleansing. Recent studies suggest that it contains similar chemicals to devil's claw so could also be helpful for arthritic conditions as an anti-inflammatory.
Actions: cleansing, diuretic, laxative, anti-inflammatory, wound herb, lymphatic cleanser, heart stimulant
Caution: avoid in tachycardia (rapid heart beat)

Garlic (*Allium sativum*)—familiar as a food flavouring, garlic has been used for treating colds and catarrh since ancient Egyptian times. Modern research has also confirmed its role in treating heart and circulatory problems.
Actions: antibiotic, expectorant, diaphoretic, hypotensive, reduces blood clotting, reduces cholesterol and blood sugar levels, antihistamine, anti-parasitic
Caution: can irritate weak stomachs and sensitive skins. Avoid high doses in pregnancy and breast-feeding

Ginger—see Chapter 5

Ginkgo (*Ginkgo biloba*)—grown in many botanical gardens as an ornamental since 1727. It is a deciduous conifer—a rare fossil survivor. Recent research has demonstrated that it will significantly improve cerebral circulation and it is now used for a wide range of blood disorders. In traditional Chinese medicine it is recommended for asthma and urinary problems.
Actions: Leaves: vasodilator, circulatory stimulant, anti-inflammatory; seeds: astringent, anti-fungal, anti-bacterial

Ginseng (*Panax ginseng*)—used in China for more than 5,000 years and believed to strengthen the body's vital energy (*Qi*). The plant is rich in steroidal compounds which are very similar to human sex hormones; hence its reputation as an aphrodisiac. It is, however, a rather more all-round tonic, helping the body adapt to stressful situations and especially valuable for the elderly and to strengthen the lungs. As a general tonic it is ideally taken for a month in late autumn when the weather is changing from hot summer to cold winter and the body needs to adapt to the new environment.

Actions: tonic, stimulant, reduces blood sugar and cholesterol levels, immunostimulant

Caution: do not take for more than four weeks without a break; avoid taking with caffeine and in pregnancy

Golden seal (*Hydrastis canadensis*)—once used by the Cherokee for digestive problems and to make an insect-repellent ointment. The root has a bitter taste and acts as a digestive stimulant but the plant will also combat infections and is useful for catarrh and hay fever. It can ease hot flushes at the menopause.

Actions: astringent, tonic, anti-inflammatory, bitter, digestive and bile stimulant, anti-catarrhal, laxative, healing to gastric mucosa, may increase blood pressure, uterine stimulant

Caution: avoid in pregnancy and high blood pressure

Gotu kola (*Centella asiatica*)—an Ayurvedic tonic herb long used as a rejuvenating remedy to counter the problems of old age and improve failing memory. In the West it has been used to speed post-operative recovery, for skin disorders and rheumatism.

Actions: tonic, anti-rheumatic, peripheral vasodilator, diuretic, sedative, bitter, laxative

Gugulla (*Boswellia serrata*)—an Indian variety of frankincense, *gugulla* is traditionally used as an anti-inflammatory remedy given for a wide range of conditions including inflammatory bowel disease, asthma, allergic rhinitis, urticaria and psoriasis as well as gout and rheumatoid arthritis.

Actions: anti-inflammatory, anti-arthritic, reduces cholesterol levels

Hawthorn (*Crataegus laevigata; C. monogyna*)—widely used as a cardiac tonic and will improve peripheral circulation, regulate heart rate and blood pressure and improve coronary blood flow. As an astringent it was more often used in the past for sore throats and diarrhoea.

Actions: cardiotonic, vasodilator, relaxant, anti-spasmodic, regulates blood pressure, diuretic

Heartsease (*Viola tricolor*)—a popular garden flower that is good for coughs, bronchitis and whooping cough, and can soothe skin inflammations and eczema. It is rich in flavonoids (including rutin) so will strengthen capillary walls. Heartsease infusion can be used as a wash to bath skin sores, nappy rash and cradle cap.
Actions: expectorant, anti-inflammatory, diuretic, anti-rheumatic, laxative, stabilises capillary membranes

Huang Bai (*Phellodendron amurense*)—first recorded in 1578 in the great herbal of Li Shi Zhen—a contemporary of John Gerard in England. The Chinese name translates as 'yellow fir' and the herb is an important remedy for clearing heat and damp and detoxifying. It is included in remedies for some types of *Bi Zheng*.
Actions: anti-bacterial, hypotensive, lowers blood sugar, cholagogue, diuretic
Caution: avoid in diarrhoea or for those with weak stomachs

Jasmine—see Chapter 5

Juniper—see Chapter 5

Lavender—see Chapter 5

Lemon—see Chapter 5

Lemon balm (*Melissa officinalis*)—associated by the ancient Greeks with bees and the healing power of honey (hence its botanical name), lemon balm is a gentle herb useful for treating nervous tummy upsets in children but also potent enough to help with depression, anxiety and tension headaches. Externally, lemon balm creams can be used on insect bites, sores and slow-healing wounds. The essential oil, known as melissa oil, is calming and restorative and especially helpful for dealing with the shock of severe illness.

Actions: sedative, anti-depressant, digestive stimulant, peripheral vasodilator, diaphoretic, relaxing restorative for nervous system, anti-viral, anti-bacterial

Lime (*Tilia cordata*)—a popular after-dinner tisane in France taken to encourage relaxation as well as improve the digestion after eating. The plant is calming for the nerves and can help to reduce high blood pressure. It is believed to combat the build up of fatty deposits in the blood vessels that can lead to atherosclerosis.
Actions: anti-spasmodic, diaphoretic, diuretic, sedative, anti-coagulant, immune stimulant, digestive remedy

Lobelia (*Lobelia inflata*)—known as pukeweed in its native America, lobelia is a potent emetic popular in the days of heroic medicine. It is mainly used as an anti-spasmodic and relaxant, helpful in conditions like asthma. It can be useful externally in creams to ease muscle cramps and spasm.
Actions: anti-spasmodic, mild sedative, relaxant, expectorant, dia-phoretic, broncho-dilator, emetic, respiratory stimulant
Caution: avoid in weakness and debility, in pregnancy or shock; high doses cause vomiting

Marigold (*Calendula officinalis*)—familiar in patent 'calendula creams' used for dry skin and eczema, the herb is also a powerful menstrual regulator and digestive remedy. As an anti-fungal it is helpful for vaginal thrush and athlete's foot; it is also detoxifying and helpful in chronic infections.
Actions: astringent, antiseptic, anti-fungal, anti-inflammatory, anti-spasmodic, wound herb, menstrual regulator, immune stimulator, diaphoretic, oestrogenic

Marjoram—see Chapter 5

Milk thistle (*Silybum marianum*)—usually regarded as a protec-tive remedy for the liver. It contains silymarin which has been shown to prevent toxic chemicals from damaging the liver and has also been successfully used for liver cirrhosis and hepatitis.

Formerly the plant was used to encourage milk flow in nursing mothers—hence its name.

Actions: bitter tonic, protects the liver, stimulates bile flow, increases milk flow, anti-depressant, anti-viral

Monkshood (*Aconitum napellus*)—restricted in the UK to external use by practitioners only, monkshood is a poison although it was used internally as a heart remedy in the past. Herbalists like Rudolf Weiss (1988) suggest it internally with autumn crocus for the pain of arthritis and gout. Externally it can relieve the pain of facial and intercostal neuralgia, rheumatism, lumbago and arthritis and can be used in liniments (1ml of tincture to 100ml of witch hazel) or compresses. Related species are used in Chinese medicine for arthritis and rheumatic disorders.

Actions: slows heart beat, anti-bacterial, anti-viral, anti-fungal

Caution: do not take internally; for professional use only

Parsley (*Petroselinum crispum*)—more familiar as a garnish, parsley is also a valuable medicinal herb and is a good source of vitamins and minerals. It is often used as a diuretic for premenstrual fluid retention and is a cleansing remedy in rheumatism. Chewing fresh parsley reputedly reduces the lingering smell of garlic.

Actions: anti-spasmodic, anti-rheumatic, diuretic, carminative, expectorant, tonic, anti-microbial, nutrient

Caution: avoid therapeutic doses in pregnancy

Passion flower (*Passiflora incarnata*)—takes its name from the religious symbolism of its flowers rather than any therapeutic effects. It was traditionally used by Native Americans as a tonic and remedy for epilepsy. Today it is regarded as an effective, but gentle sedative largely used for insomnia.

Actions: sedative, anti-spasmodic, vasodilator, analgesic, tranquilliser

Caution: avoid high doses in pregnancy; may cause drowsiness

Peppermint—see Chapter 5

Pine—see Chapter 5

Psyllium seeds (*Plantago psyllium; P. ovata*)—also known as ispaghula, psyllium is widely used as a bulking laxative: the seeds swell when moistened to form a glutinous mass which encourages peristalsis and lubricates the bowel. Although primarily used for constipation, the resulting bulky mass can help to soothe diarrhoea and is sometimes recommended in irritable bowel syndrome.
Actions: demulcent, bulk laxative, anti-diarrhoeal
Caution: always take capsules or dried psyllium with plenty of water to avoid excess absorption of stomach fluids

Qin Jiao (*Gentiana macrophylla*)—used for wind–damp types of *Bi Zheng* in traditional Chinese medicine, *Qin Jiao* is also used to clear heat–damp. The plant is known in English as large-leaved gentian and has been used in TCM for at least 2,000 years.
Actions: anti-bacterial, anti-inflammatory, analgesic, sedative, increases blood sugar, lowers blood pressure
Caution: avoid in polyuria (frequent urination), diarrhoea or debility

Red clover (*Trifolium pratense*)—mainly used by herbalists as a cleansing remedy for skin problems such as psoriasis and eczema. It is a useful expectorant and diuretic helpful for dry coughs and gout, while the fresh flowers can relieve insect bites and stings. The herb was used in the 1930s in cancer therapy and still finds a role in the treatment of breast and skin cancers.
Actions: cleansing, anti-spasmodic, diuretic, possible oestrogenic activity

Reishi mushroom (*Ganoderma lucidem*)—the reishi mushroom was highly regarded by the ancient Chinese Taoists as a spiritual tonic and one which could enhance longevity. The herb is now known to stimulate the immune system so can be valuable for recurrent infections and debility. It has been used for chronic fatigue syndrome, ME and AIDS.
Actions: reduces blood pressure and cholesterol levels, anti-viral, immune-stimulant, expectorant, anti-tussive, antihistamine, anti-tumour

St John's wort (*Hypericum perforatum*)—a traditional wound herb and pain remedy, St John's wort is now becoming better known as an anti-depressant and is widely prescribed by German doctors. It has also been used in AIDS treatments and is a valuable external remedy for minor burns and grazes.
Actions: astringent, analgesic, anti-inflammatory, sedative, restoring tonic for the nervous system, anti-depressant, anti-spasmodic, anti-viral
Caution: prolonged use may increase the photosensitivity of the skin and may lead to cornea damage; recent studies suggest it might interfere with the action of other drugs so should not be taken with prescription medicines without professional advice

Shatavari (*Asparagus racemosus*)—a close relative of our familiar Western vegetable, Asian asparagus is one of Ayurveda's most important tonics. It is used for any debility associated with the female sexual organs including infertility, menopausal problems and following hysterectomy. It is also regarded as a soothing demulcent for the digestive and respiratory systems used for dry coughs, fevers associated with thirst, pleurisy, sunstroke, and inflammatory digestive problems such as dysentery.
Actions: tonic, demulcent, antibacterial, anti-tussive, expectorant, anti-tumour
Cautions: traditionally avoided in cases of diarrhoea and coughs caused by common colds

Shiitake mushroom (*Lentinula edodes*)—now familiar on supermarket shelves the shiitake mushroom is an important immune stimulant and tonic. Extracts of the mushroom have been used in Japan to help support patients undergoing chemotherapy and it has been shown to reduce the growth rate of liver tumours; in the USA it has been used for AIDS sufferers and is believed to improve the immune and endocrine function in the elderly. The mushroom has featured in traditional Chinese medicine for at least 2,000 years.
Actions: anti-viral, anti-tumour, lowers cholesterol levels, immune stimulant, liver tonic

Siberian ginseng (*Eleutherococcus senticosus*)—came to fame in the 1950s when it was extensively used by Soviet athletes to increase stamina and enhance performance. The herb's main application is as a tonic, helping the body to cope with increased stress levels and to provide extra energy.
Actions: tonic, stimulant, combats stress, anti-viral, lowers blood sugar, immune stimulant
Caution: do not exceed standard dose (usually 600mg daily) or take for prolonged periods

Skullcap (*Scutellaria lateriflora*)—originally found in Virginia, this variety of skullcap was introduced into Europe in the 18th century as a treatment for rabies. Today, it is mainly used as a relaxing sedative for stress and anxiety, although in the past it was recommended for jaundice, urinary tract infections, haemorrhage and threatened miscarriage.
Actions: relaxing and restorative nervine, anti-spasmodic, bitter

Slippery elm (*Ulmus rubra*)—a highly mucilaginous herb mainly used to coat the stomach and provide protection in cases of gastritis, heartburn and ulceration. It is also a valuable nutrient which can be made into a gruel with hot milk and flavoured with honey and spices for convalescents or the seriously debilitated. Externally it makes an effective drawing ointment for splinters and boils and can also soothe wounds and burns.
Actions: demulcent, emollient, laxative, nutritive, anti-tussive

Sweet flag (*Acorus calamus*)—important in Ayurvedic medicine as a rejuvenating tonic for the nervous system, sweet flag is mainly used in the West as a digestive remedy to ease abdominal bloating and colic and normalise function. The plant has been used in China for rheumatoid arthritis.
Actions: carminative, diaphoretic, anti-spasmodic, digestive stimulant, bitter, anti-tussive, lowers blood pressure, anti-bacterial
Caution: some varieties contain asarone, which is carcinogenic; take for short periods only under professional guidance. Restricted in some countries

Thyme—see Chapter 5

Valerian (*Valeriana officinalis*)—one of the most popular herbal sedatives, used for anxiety and insomnia. It also reduces high blood pressure and is sometimes recommended for a range of heart conditions. It is totally non-addictive and helpful for many stress-related disorders. Extracts are sometimes used in skin creams for eczema.
Actions: tranquilliser, anti-spasmodic, expectorant, diuretic, hypotensive, carminative, mild anodyne
Caution: excess may cause headache; do not combine with sleep-enhancing drugs

Vervain (*Verbena officinalis*)—a sacred herb to both Romans and Druids and continued to be associated with magic and fortune-telling until well into the 17th century. Today it is valued as a useful nervine and liver tonic. It is bitter and stimulating for the digestion and makes an ideal tonic in convalescence and debility. Externally it can ease the pain of neuralgia.
Actions: relaxant tonic, stimulates milk production, diaphoretic, nervine, sedative, anti-spasmodic, hepatic restorative, laxative, uterine stimulant, bile stimulant
Caution: avoid in pregnancy, although it can be taken in labour to stimulate contractions

Wild yam (*Dioscorea villosa*)—the original source of the oral contraceptive pill as it is rich in steroidal saponins. It is largely used for colic and rheumatism but can also be taken for period pain, cramps, asthma, gastritis and gall bladder problems.
Actions: Relaxant for smooth muscle, anti-spasmodic, stimulates bile flow, anti-inflammatory, mild diaphoretic
Caution: May cause nausea in high doses

Wintergreen —see Chapter 5

White poplar (*Populus tremuloides*)—like white willow, a rich source of salicylate-like compounds with an extensive history of use as a remedy for arthritis and rheumatic disorders; the plant can also be used for reducing fevers. Often used as an alternative to white willow or meadowsweet.

Actions: anti-rheumatic, antiseptic, anti-inflammatory, mild analgesic, febrifuge, tonic, stimulant

Caution: avoid in aspirin or salicylate allergy

Witch-hazel (*Hamamelis virginiana*)—a first-aid standby. Virginian witch hazel was used by many North American tribes: the Menomees rubbed the decoction into their legs to keep them supple during sports, while the Potawatomis put witch hazel twigs into sweat baths to relieve sore muscles. It is usually supplied as a distillate for external use, ideal in rubs for relieving muscle strains, joint sprains and bruises. Internally it is taken for diarrhoea, colitis, excessive menstruation and haemorrhage.

Actions: astringent, stops internal and external bleeding, anti-inflammatory

Yarrow (*Achillea millefolium*)—a common meadow herb used in remedies for colds, hay fever and catarrh. As a diuretic, it can also be used for urinary problems, in cleansing mixtures and to counter fluid retention or reduce blood pressure. The essential oil is very similar to chamomile in action and can be used for joint and tendon inflammations such as tennis elbow in the same way.

Actions: Aerial parts/flowers—astringent, diaphoretic, peripheral vasodilator, digestive stimulant, restorative for menstrual system, febrifuge. Essential oil—anti-inflammatory, anti-allergenic, anti-spasmodic

Caution: a uterine stimulant, so avoid in pregnancy; the fresh plant can sometimes cause contact dermatitis and, rarely, may increase the skin's photosensitivity

Yellow dock (*Rumex crispus*)—a cleansing herb suitable for chronic skin problems and arthritic complaints. It helps to clear toxins and acts as a gentle stimulant for liver and kidneys. It can also be used as a blood tonic in anaemia and is a lymphatic cleanser, useful for swollen glands. It is an astringent remedy and can be used for wounds.

Actions: laxative, bile stimulant, cleansing
Caution: avoid regular use or high doses in pregnancy and lactation

Yellow jasmine (*Gelsemium sempervirens*)—restricted to practitioner use in the UK, yellow jasmine is a powerful relaxant for the central nervous system and an analgesic. It can be used to relieve neuralgia, cramp and back pains and is also helpful for nervous headaches and migraine.
Actions: nerve relaxant, vasodilator, analgesic, anti-spasmodic, tranquilliser
Caution: not for home use; may be prescribed by qualified practitioners only

Yi Yi Ren (*Coix lachryma-jobi*)—Job's tear seeds (*Yi Yi Ren*) can be used in cooking rather like pearl barley for making porridge and soups. The herb has a wide range of uses in Chinese medicine: it is a digestive remedy, used to regulate water metabolism, stop diarrhoea and clear inflammations. It also clears wind–damp which can lead to 'painful obstructions' and *Bi Zheng* (arthritis-like symptoms).
Actions: muscle relaxant, anti-tumour, analgesic, sedative, lowers blood sugar, anti-pyretic
Caution: avoid in pregnancy

Zhi Mu (*Anemarrhena asphodeloides*)—a type of night-flowering lily, *Zhi Mu* is used in Chinese medicine for lower back pains and feverish conditions which may be associated with excess heat and fire in the system. It is known to contain steroidal compounds.
Actions: anti-bacterial, anti-fungal, anti-pyretic, expectorant, diuretic, lowers blood sugar
Caution: high doses may cause breathing difficulties and irregular heart beat

CHAPTER 5

Aromatic Remedies

Aromatic oils have been used for centuries to make soothing balms for aching joints and muscles. Externally, herbs which encourage blood flow to the skin (rubefacients) are often applied in poultices; in the past the aim would be to encourage blistering (seen as the visible removal of toxins) although modern medicine takes a less robust approach to treatment.

The essence or essential oil is most commonly collected by steam distillation: the plant material is heated over a water bath so that steam rises through the herb and dissolves the highly volatile oils. This distillate is then condensed in a cooler and collected. The oil, being lighter than water, floats to the surface and is easily skimmed off. Essential oils are thus a highly concentrated plant extract and can be extremely potent.

Although technically quite simple steam distillation is not a technique for home use—many tonnes of leaves and flowering tops are needed to produce viable commercial quantities of oil. Yields are typically 0.1–10%—it takes 2,000kg of rose petals, for example, to produce just one kilo of rose oil.

Although in parts of Europe, notably France, essential oils are prescribed for internal use, in the UK they are almost always used in external treatments: mostly in well-diluted massage rubs by aromatherapists, added to baths or sometimes used in steam inhalants for nasal congestion. Until fairly recently British aromatherapy was considered by many as more of a relaxing type of beauty treatment than a reputable medical therapy. Essential oils are very potent medicine and using them—even in dilute mixtures—purely as a beauty aid is both dangerous and misleading.

Today, aromatherapy and relaxing massage are among the most

popular complementary therapies. Many of the oils used in such treatments have significant anti-inflammatory and analgesic action so can be especially effective for muscle strains, pains or arthritic disorders.

Using Oils for Aches and Pains

For home use it is best to limit the essential oils to external massage, lotions, inhalants or baths: internal use needs skill and experience and is not recommended unless under professional guidance.

While professional therapists may sometimes used concentrated oils, they really should be kept very dilute for home use. Typically massage rubs are not more than 5% oil (up to 5ml or 100 drops with 95ml of carrier oil, such as almond or wheatgerm) and often may contain as little as 1%, while only 5–10 drops of oil need be added to bath water. Some oils are used by herbalists in higher concentrations: 20% is not unusual for lavender or rosemary. A few drops of oil can also be added to simple skin creams or dispersed in a little vodka or distilled witch hazel to make a lotion or spray.

Oils can be used singly or in combinations and mixed either in a plain vegetable-oil base (such as wheatgerm or almond oil) or used with an infused oil. These can be made using either the hot infusion or cold infusion methods.

Hot infusion: this is used for leaves such as comfrey. Heat 100g of dried (300g fresh) herb in 500ml of sunflower oil (or similar) in a double saucepan over water for about three hours. Remember to refill the lower saucepan with hot water from time to time to prevent it from boiling dry. After about three hours the oil will take on a greenish colour. Strain the mix through a sieve, muslin bag or wine press and store in clean glass bottles, away from direct sunlight.

Some herbs, such as bladderwrack (see Chapter 4), which is especially good for arthritic pain and swellings, need more vigorous treatment. Use 500g of dried bladderwrack to 500ml of sunflower oil and leave to soak overnight, then bring to the boil and simmer for 20 minutes. Strain the mixture while still warm.

Cold infusion: this method is ideal for flowering tips, such as

St John's wort. Because the oil is not heated in this method, good-quality seed oils that are rich in essential fatty acids (EFA)— such as *gamma*-linolenic or *cis*-linoleic (see Chapter 7)—can be used; these have significant therapeutic properties and add to the potency of the infused oil mixture. Oils high in EFA include walnut, safflower and pumpkin oils. Fill a large clear glass jar with flowers and cover completely with oil. This is important as any herb exposed to the air may go mouldy and the mixture will be spoilt. Leave the jar on a sunny window-sill or in the greenhouse for at least three weeks and then strain and store the mixture as with hot infused oils.

Massage Mixtures and Baths

Mixed massage oils soon deteriorate so are best made in small quantities (e.g. 20ml) and stored in dark glass bottles. Use about half a teaspoon (2.5ml) at a time and massage the affected area gently; vigorous massage can be damaging for some conditions, especially gout and types of arthritis.

Essential oils can also be added neat to bath water: stir the water vigorously before getting into the bath as concentrated drops of the oil can have an unpleasant effect on sensitive skin.

Arthritis
- For osteoarthritis add 2ml of rosemary oil to 18ml of infused comfrey oil and store in a dark glass bottle. Apply as need be to aching joints. Add five drops of benzoin and black pepper if poor circulation is a problem.
- For general joint pains use five drops each of benzoin, chamomile, juniper and rosemary in 20ml of almond or wheatgerm oil, store in a dark glass bottle and use as need be.
- For rheumatoid arthritis use 2ml of chamomile oil to 18ml of infused St John's wort oil and store in a dark glass bottle. Apply as often as need be to soothe painful joints.
- Add five drops of rosemary, benzoin and marjoram to bath water.

112

Lumbago and low back pains

- Use equal amounts of infused St John's wort oil and camphorated oil as a massage or add 5ml of the mixture to bath water.
- Add 10 drops of juniper oil and two drops of ginger or black pepper oil to 5ml of sweet almond oil and massage gently into the aching area.
- Combine 10 drops each of lavender, pine and marjoram with two drops of black pepper oil in 5ml of sweet almond oil and massage gently into the aching area.
- Add five drops each of lavender, clary sage and pine oil to bath water.

Muscular aches and pains

- Combine five drops each of thyme, lavender and marjoram oil in 20ml of almond or wheatgerm oil, store in a dark glass bottle and rub gently into the affected area night and morning.
- Combine 10 drops each of eucalyptus, rosemary and marjoram in 20ml of almond or wheatgerm oil, store in a dark glass bottle and use as need be.

Muscle stiffness

- Massage with two drops of black pepper oil in 2.5ml (half a teaspoon) of almond or infused cayenne or nettle oil.
- Combine 10 drops each of rosemary, clary sage and marjoram oils in 20ml of almond or infused cayenne oil, store in a dark glass bottle and use as need be.

Rheumatic aches and pains

- Combine five drops each of juniper, cypress and clary sage oil in 20ml of almond or infused comfrey oil, store in a dark glass bottle and use as need be.
- Add two–three drops of juniper oils to bath water.
- Bartram (1995) recommends wintergreen liniment as an invigorating rub for rheumatic aches. Mix 20 drops of

wintergreen oil, 10 drops of peppermint oil, and five drops of camphor with 25g (1oz) soft soap and 100g (4oz) alcohol. Shake before use and rub into aching muscles as need be.

Sciatica

- Combine 10 drops each of pine, lavender and chamomile oils in 20ml of infused St John's wort oil, store in a dark glass bottle and use as need be.
- Add five drops of pine and lavender oil to bath water.

Sprains and strains

- Combine 10 drops of lavender and 10 drops of chamomile with 500ml of cold water. Use to soak a compress and apply to the damaged area. Alternate the cold compress with a hot compress made by soaking a cotton cloth in boiling water containing 10 drops of rosemary and five drops of black pepper oils.

Tendinitis, tenosynovitis and bursa problems

- For conditions like tennis elbow, mix 20 drops of chamomile or yarrow oil and 20 drops of benzoin oil in 20ml of infused St John's wort oil, store in a dark glass bottle and rub gently into the affected area several times a day.

Aromatic Chemistry

Essential oils contain a complex cocktail of organic chemicals. There may be dozens in any one oil and in many cases they have not all been fully identified. These aromatic carbon-based compounds are classified by their structure and oxygen content— such as alcohols, ketones, aldehydes, phenols, acids and esters (Table 3). In plants the basic molecular building block is a group of five linked carbon atoms (C_5); these build up to form large molecules known as terpenes—monoterpenes (C_{10}), sesquiterpenes (C_{15}), and diterpenes (C_{20}). Terpenes are compounds containing carbon (C) and hydrogen (H) while terpenoids also contain oxygen

Table 3: Categories of simple chemical constituents

Group	Structure	Examples
Alcohols	R—OH	linalol (lavender); borneol (rosemary)
Aldehydes	$\begin{array}{c} R \\ \diagdown \\ H \end{array} C = O$	citral (ginger)
Ketones	$\begin{array}{c} R \\ \diagdown \\ R^1 \end{array} C = O$	carvone (caraway); thujone (sage)
Epoxides	$\begin{array}{c} -C \\ \mid \\ -C \end{array} \diagdown O$	cineole (Spanish sage)
Phenols	OH	eugenol (clove); thymol (thyme)
Esters	R—COOR^1	linalyl acetate (lavender)
Acids	R—COOH	citric acid (*Citrus* spp.); rosmarinic acid (rosemary)

NB: R and R^1 represent alkyl groups such as CH_3-(methyl); C_2H_5-(ethyl) etc.

(O). The aromatic compounds found in essential oils are mainly terpenoids.

In general aromatic aldehydes tend to be antiseptic, alcohols are tonic and stimulating, and ketones are usually toxic (Gattefossé, 1937). Since the 1930s, French aromatherapists have tried to classify these various groups of chemicals in terms of electrical energy—positive or negative—which phytotherapists like Pierre Franchomme (1985) equate with *yang* or *yin* activity. Negative or *yin* compounds are more passive, gentle and inwardly focusing while the *yang* chemicals are more active, aggressive, and out-wardly moving. Franchomme sees aldehydes and esters as more *yin* in character, while alcohols and monoterpenes have a *yang* bias, with ketones in between.

For 'cold' conditions such as rheumatic pains, muscular stiffness and osteoarthritis, warming or *yang* constituents are best, while for inflammatory disorders, such as tendinitis or rheumatoid arthritis, cooling or *yin* oils are preferable.

Key Essential Oils Index

Benzoin
Botanical name: *Styrax benzoin*
Actions: anti-inflammatory, antioxidant, antiseptic, astringent, carminative, diuretic, expectorant, sedative, styptic, wound herb
Extraction: crude benzoin is collected directly from the trees as an exuded balsamic resin which hardens with exposure to air and sunlight; this is then purified using solvents such as benzene and alcohol. Commercial benzoin is generally sold dissolved in ethyl glycol or other similar solvents

Benzoin is most familiar in a compound tincture form known as Friars Balsam and popularly used for respiratory complaints. It was a traditional ingredient in incense, used to drive out evil spirits. Today it is mainly regarded as warming and stimulating to help energise digestive function, elimination and the circulation. It can be helpful where joint or muscle pains are associated with sluggish metabolism or poor circulation.

Birch
Botanical name: *Betula* spp.
Actions: analgesic, anti-inflammatory, anti-pyretic, anti-rheumatic, antiseptic, astringent, depurative, diuretic, rubefacient, tonic
Extraction: by steam distillation of the bark after soaking in warm water

Oil extracted from the North American sweet (*B. lenta*) and yellow (*B. alleghaniensis*) birch trees are around 98% methyl salicylate and are chemically almost identical to oil of wintergreen; indeed much of the oil sold as birch is actually synthetic methyl salicylate. This chemical was first identified in willow trees and related chemicals are the basis of aspirin. Like other salicylates birch oil is analgesic, anti-spasmodic and anti-inflammatory and is a traditional remedy for all sorts of rheumatic and arthritic aches and pains as well as muscle cramps and tendinitis.

In aromatherapy it is sometimes used in massage mixtures for muscular pains and is also a cleansing remedy so helps elimination of toxins. The oil can also help remove uric acid from joints so can be valuable in gouty conditions (Franchomme and Penoel, 1991; Veal, 1998).

European birch oil (*B. pendula*) is also used for treating rheumatism although chemically it is very different from the North American variety. It contains a mixture of phenols and is also an effective disinfectant for skin conditions.

Birch oil is also produced from *B. alba* and is mainly used as a hair and skin remedy. This oil is most often available commercially and can be confused with the North American oil used for joint and muscle pains. Some authorities (Viaud, 1983) suggest that *B. alba* can be carcinogenic and should be avoided but there seems little firm evidence for this, although since it contains no methyl salicylate it is unlikely to be very effective for treating muscular aches and pains anyway.

In European herbal tradition, infusions of birch leaf are used for rheumatoid arthritis and gout and various proprietary birch elixirs are marked in Germany and Switzerland as arthritic remedies. The plant is believed to work on purine metabolism in some as yet little-understood way.

Caution: methyl salicylate is extremely toxic in large doses and can cause blistering of the skin; it should be used in very weak dilution (around 2%) in massage therapy. Like all salicylates it should be avoided by those taking warfarin and similar blood-thinning drugs

Black pepper
Botanical name: *Piper nigrum*
Actions: analgesic, anti-microbial, antiseptic, anti-spasmodic, aphrodisiac, anti-bacterial, carminative, diaphoretic, digestive, diuretic, febrifuge, laxative, rubefacient, stimulant, tonic
Extraction: by steam distillation of black peppercorns which have been dried and crushed

Black pepper has been used as a culinary seasoning in Europe since at least the fifth century and has been known in the East for around 4,000 years. The essential oil mainly contains monoterpenes (70–80%) and sesquiterpenes which suggest that it can also help strengthen the immune system and the remedy is a traditional standby for colds and infections.

Black pepper is very warming and stimulating and is often used in aromatherapy for digestive problems and also to stimulate the kidneys. Its main use is in aromatic rubs for muscular aches and pains as well as stiffness and fatigue. It is rubefacient, which means it will draw blood to the surface and so can be used to warm a particular area. The oil needs to be used only in small quantities as it can be an irritant.

Aromatherapists like Patricia Davis (1995) recommend black pepper oil for use in massage rubs for dancers and athletes as it can help combat pain and stiffness and, apparently, improve performance as well.

Cayenne
Botanical name: *Capsicum frutescens*
Actions: circulatory stimulant, tonic, anti-spasmodic, diaphoretic, gastric stimulant, carminative, antiseptic, anti-bacterial, analgesic. Use topically as a counter-irritant and rubefacient.
Extraction: infused cayenne oil—rather than an extracted essential oil—is used. This is made by simmering 25g (1oz) of dried cayenne (use the whole dried fruits coarsely ground rather than commercial powder if possible) with 500ml of sunflower oil for two hours over a water bath

Chilli, or cayenne, has become familiar in sauces and flavourings in recent years thanks to growing interest in Oriental and West Indian cookery. The herb first arrived in Britain from India in the 1540s and was known as 'ginnie pepper'. The Elizabethan herbalist, John Gerard, was less than enthusiastic about its properties, declaring that it was an 'enemie of the liver' and would also 'killeth dogs'. He did, however, recommend it for scrofula—a prevalent lymphatic throat and skin infection known as the King's Evil and reputedly healed by the touch of a reigning monarch.

Various chilli species are used medicinally including *C. frutescens* and the hot pepper used in cooking, *C. annuum*. Chilli became extremely popular in the 19th century with the Physiomedicalists, a group of traditional healers originating in 18th-century New England where the icy winters certainly brought plenty of colds and chills to be warmed by spicy herbs.

The herb is diaphoretic so increases perspiration; as such it was used in the 'sweating' treatments favoured by these 19th-century healers, which were based on the Native American tradition of sweat lodges. Many Western herbalists still add chilli to mixtures for treating such 'cold' complaints as arthritis, digestive weakness and general debility and the herb is regarded as a useful stimulant both for the digestion and circulation.

Externally, cayenne ointments can be used to encourage blood flow and may be used for treating chilblains, lumbago, muscle pain, the pain of shingles, and nerve pains like neuralgia.

Caution: avoid in stomach ulceration, pregnancy and breast-feeding. Do not eat seeds on their own and avoid touching eyes or cuts after handling fresh chilli.

Chamomile
Botanical name: *Matricaria recutita/Chamaemelum nobile*
Actions: anti-inflammatory, anti-spasmodic, bitter, sedative, carminative, anti-emetic, anti-allergenic
Extraction: by steam distillation of the flowers

Both German chamomile (*Matricaria recutita*) and its relative Roman chamomile (*Chamaemelum nobile*) are used in aroma-

119

therapy. German chamomile oil is a distinctive inky-blue colour while Roman chamomile is a pale blue fading to a straw colour with storage. Just as the flowers are used in very similar ways by herbalists, so too with the oils although their chemical composition is quite different.

German chamomile is largely made up of chamazulene—responsible for the blue colour. This is an anti-allergenic and anti-inflammatory chemical and makes the oil especially useful for conditions like hay fever or allergic asthma as well as inflammatory joint problems. Roman chamomile is mainly made up of esters so is calming and sedating with less focus on anti-inflammatory action.

Like the flowers, however, the oils are used almost interchangeably in massage treatments for skin and digestive problems, to ease menstrual and menopausal discomfort, and as a urinary antiseptic in conditions such as cystitis.

Anti-inflammatory German chamomile oil can be especially helpful for acute inflammations such as tennis elbow or tendinitis. **Caution**: the fresh plant can cause contact dermatitis in sensitive individuals

Clary sage
Botanical name: *Salvia sclarea*
Actions: anti-bacterial, anti-convulsive, anti-depressant, antiseptic, anti-spasmodic, aphrodisiac, astringent, carminative, deodorant, digestive, emmenagogue, hypotensive, nervine, seborrhoeic regulator, sedative, tonic, uterine stimulant
Extraction: by steam distillation of the flowering tops and leaves. The yield can be as low as 0.05% which makes it difficult to produce, so good-quality oil can be expensive

Clary sage is a popular essence in the perfumery market, used in scents and soaps, while its muscatel flavour makes it valuable as a food essence and it is often used in the drinks industry to flavour wines.

The plant is rich in esters so that it is primarily rebalancing and anti-spasmodic. It is ideal for combating both depression and over-excitability and it works at a deep level acting as a restorative for emotional and spiritual problems. Clary sage oil is also excellent for gynaecological problems such as amenorrhoea, dysmenorrhoea, and vaginal discharges (leucorrhoea). It can be an appropriate choice at the menopause to combat depression.

It is often used for back pains as a muscle relaxant and it can be ideal in baths before bedtime as the oil is very calming and relaxing, leading to drowsiness and sleep.

Clary sage oil is generally regarded as mildly hypotensive to reduce blood pressure (Rovesti and Gattefossé, 1973). It will also stimulate the adrenal cortex so may be helpful for those recovering from a course of steroidal therapy.

Caution: avoid clary sage oil in pregnancy and when drinking alcohol as it can enhance the effect. Avoid driving after using clary sage in massage treatments

Comfrey
Botanical name: *Symphytum officinale*
Actions: astringent, demulcent, expectorant, tissue healer and cell proliferant
Extraction: the infused oil is used, prepared by the hot infusion method (see above)

Although comfrey has been used for centuries as a wound healer and restorer of broken bones—its country name is 'knitbone' and the botanical name is derived from the Greek *sympho*, meaning to unite—it has had a more chequered history in recent years, veering from panacea to health hazard.

Its healing action is due to a chemical called allantoin which encourages growth of various tissue cells and so accelerates healing. Generations used comfrey poultices on pulled ligaments and minor fractures, while herbalists used it internally for stomach ulceration. The immense healing properties of the plant have been put to many diverse uses over the centuries: in the past comfrey baths were popular before marriage in the belief that they would repair the hymen and thus create the appearance of virginity.

During the 1960s and 1970s the plant became over-hyped as a

cure-all for arthritis and this inevitably focused research interest on its constituents. Scientists fed large amounts of the plant to rats which subsequently died of liver disease, and comfrey's pyrrolizidine alkaloids were blamed. Comfrey supporters argue that the rats had so much comfrey to eat they actually suffered from the effects of malnutrition and maintain that the alkaloids are not in fact extracted in conventional herbal preparations (infusions and ointments). Health authorities have tended to disagree and comfrey is now banned in many parts of the world. In the UK the leaf can still be sold over the counter and it can be used in external preparations although many advise against using it on open wounds.

The hot infused oil is easy to make and forms a useful base for massage oils for arthritis, sprains and similar traumatic injuries. Regular treatment can help repair the damage of old injuries which many be contributing to osteoarthritis and it is extremely healing for any sort of bruising.

Caution: the dangers of pyrrolizidine alkaloids apart, the herb should not be used on fresh wounds before they are thoroughly cleaned since the rapid healing caused by the allantoin may trap dirt, so leading to abscesses

Cypress

Botanical name: *Cupresses sempervirens*

Actions: anti-rheumatic, antiseptic, anti-spasmodic, astringent, deodorant, diuretic, hepatic, styptic, tonic, peripheral vaso-constrictor

Extraction: steam distillation of the needles, cones and twigs

Cypress oil was used in incense and rituals in many ancient cultures and is still used for purification rituals in Tibet. The oil has a smoky, woody smell slightly reminiscent of turpentine and contains a mixture of aromatic terpenes including pinene, camphene and cymene.

It is mainly used in aromatherapy for urinary problems, excess menstruation and fluid retention and is also added to chest rubs and inhalants for asthma and bronchitis. Cypress oil can help stimulate the circulation and is good for relieving muscle cramps as well as rheumatic aches.

Eucalyptus
Botanical name: *Eucalyptus globulus*
Actions: antiseptic, anti-viral, anti-fungal, anti-spasmodic, stimulant, reduces fevers, hypoglycaemic
Extraction: by steam distillation of the fresh and partially dried leaves and young twigs

Originally an Aboriginal remedy, eucalyptus arrived in Europe in the 19th century and has been used as a potent antiseptic for infections ever since. The oil is mainly cyneol (up to 85%) with pinene, limonene and other terpenes.

Eucalyptus is used in aromatherapy for treating respiratory problems, such as asthma and bronchitis; it is used too for debility and nervous exhaustion and for a wide range of infectious conditions.

It makes a good rub for aching muscles and joints and is useful for rheumatoid arthritis, sprains, strains and muscle aches and pains. Eucalyptus is stimulating for the circulation so can help to warm cold joints. Fresh leaves from garden trees can be useful in inhalants and washes.

Fennel
Botanical name: *Foeniculum vulgare*
Actions: anti-inflammatory, carminative, circulatory stimulant, galactogogue, mild expectorant, diuretic
Extraction: by steam distillation of the seeds

Fennel seeds have mainly been regarded in the West as a digestive remedy to ease colic, chills and indigestion and also to stimulate milk flow in nursing mothers. The oil consists mainly of anethole (up to 60%) with limonene, pinene, camphene and various other terpenes and aldehydes.

Fennel is used in aromatherapy for digestive and respiratory problems—rather as the seeds are taken internally—and is also an effective diuretic which can be helpful for fluid retention. It helps

to clear toxic wastes from tissues so is often used by beauty therapists to combat 'cellulite', a non-medical concept associated with
fatty tissues in the limbs.

Fennel oil can also be helpful for rheumatic problems and is
useful added to treatments for muscle cramps and swelling.

Caution: avoid high doses of the herb in pregnancy; do not use
the oil in epilepsy or with children under the age of six

Ginger
Botanical name: *Zingiber officinale*
Actions: anti-emetic, anti-spasmodic, antiseptic, carminative, cir-
culatory stimulant, diaphoretic, expectorant, peripheral vaso-
dilator. Topically: rubefacient
Extraction: by steam distillation of unpeeled, dried ground root

Ginger is one of our most anti-emetic plants, helping to combat
the nausea and vomiting of both morning and motion sickness. It
is warming in chills and carminative to ease flatulence and indigestion. The oil is very warming and is used in very low dilution
(1–1.5%) to prevent skin irritation. Aromatherapists will often add
no more than a single drop to massage blends.

Ginger oil contains a mix of terpenes including gingerin,
gingenol, gingerone, linalol, borneol and citral. It can be added to
massage oils for the lower abdomen to ease digestive problems or
in chest rubs it can help with catarrh and chills—one drop on a
sugar lump is a warming remedy for colds and nausea.

As a rubefacient it can help to warm cold arthritic joints and is
also helpful where poor circulation is a factor. It is useful in
mixtures for sprains and strains, muscular aches and rheumatism.

Jasmine
Botanical name: *Jasminum officinale*
Actions: Flowers—aphrodisiac, astringent, bitter, relaxing nervine,
sedative, mild analgesic, encourages milk production. Oil—anti-
depressant, antiseptic, anti-spasmodic, aphrodisiac. Encourages
milk flow, sedative, uterine tonic. encourages parturition
Extraction: by enfleurage—a technique which involves pressing

the freshly picked flowers on to wax between two sheets of glass. The oil is extracted into the wax and then separated from it by melting the mixture. It is an expensive process and adulteration of jasmine oil with cheap synthetics is commonplace

Common jasmine is a highly aromatic climbing plant, introduced into Europe in the 16th century, which rapidly gained popularity with the French perfumiers. A close relative, royal jasmine or *jati* (*J. garndiflorum*), is an important Ayurvedic tonic and cleansing remedy. Jasmine tea, popular in China, is scented with yet another variety—*J. sambac* or Arabian jasmine, which originates in the Persian Gulf.

Jasmine oil is used in aromatherapy for period pain, anxiety and depression, impotence and frigidity, and for abdominal massage during childbirth to encourage parturition and ease labour pains. It is also added to chest rubs for coughs and breathing difficulties.

It is a good muscle relaxant so can help muscular spasms and sprains, while its uplifting effect on the nervous system helps to encourage optimism and confidence; thus it is always a good remedy to include in baths for the chronically ill and despondent.

Juniper
Botanical name: *Juniperus communis*
Actions: anti-inflammatory, anti-rheumatic, antiseptic, carminative, digestive tonic, diuretic, urinary antiseptic, uterine stimulant
Extraction: by steam distillation from either the berries or the needles and wood

Juniper berries are a favourite for flavouring game dishes. Traditionally the herb has been associated with sacred cleansing rituals and its sprigs are still regularly burned each day in Tibetan temples as part of the morning purification rite.

Juniper berries are widely used for urinary tract problems, such as cystitis, and as a cleansing remedy for rheumatism.

The essential oil is mainly composed of a mixture of monoterpenes, including pinene, myrcene, sabinene and limonene, and is used in aromatherapy for skin and urinary problems and as a stimulating tonic massage. The same oil is added as a flavouring to London gin—hence the diuretic action of that particular beverage.

Juniper berry oil is effective for clearing toxins which have accumulated in the system so is especially appropriate for gout, which is due to a build up of uric acid in the joints. It also makes a generally cleansing additive to treatments for other forms of arthritic disorders and rheumatism.

Cade oil is made by dry-distilling the heartwood of various juniper species and is used for psoriasis and other skin problems. It contains phenol and is mildly disinfectant.

Caution: prolonged use of juniper can irritate the kidneys and any preparation containing the herb should not be taken internally for longer than six weeks without professional advice; avoid completely in pregnancy and kidney disease

Lavender
Botanical name: *Lavandula angustifolia*
Actions: antiseptic, anti-bacterial, anti-depressant, carminative, relaxant, anti-spasmodic, circulatory stimulant, tonic for the nervous system, analgesic, stimulates bile flow
Extraction: by steam distillation of the flowers

Lavender has been used since Roman times as a cleansing, aromatic herb. It is valuable in herbal medicine for numerous health problems including headaches, digestive and nervous upsets. The essential oil is complex with more than 100 known ingredients including monoterpenes (such as cineol and linalol), linalyl acetate (up to 40%) and lavandulyl acetate. The exact mix varies significantly with the source of the herb.

Lavender oil is mainly used for skin problems, headaches, especially migraines, and as a relaxing sedative to combat tension and stress. It is also very effective in massage rubs to ease muscular aches and pains.

Spike lavender (*L. latifolia*) oil, sometimes sold as Spanish lavender, has quite a different mix of chemicals and is rather more penetrating and camphorous. It can be particularly effective for headaches and respiratory problems although its actions are broadly similar to those of true lavender.

A less costly alternative can be lavandin oil which is extracted from naturally occurring hybrids (*L.* X *intermedia*) mainly found in parts of Southern France. This oil is also rich in linalyl acetate but tends to be rather more camphorous than true lavender. It is used in similar ways but is particularly good for muscle stiffness after exercise or for general muscular aches and pains. Lavandin is ideal added to baths and is both analgesic and rubefacient.

Lemon
Botanical name: *Citrus limon*
Actions: anti-bacterial, anti-inflammatory, antihistamine, anti-rheumatic, anti-scorbutic, antiseptic, anti-viral, carminative, cleansing, cooling, diuretic, tonifying for heart and blood vessels
Extraction: by cold expression of the outer part of the fresh peel

Lemon was considered by the Romans to be an antidote for many poisons and in modern Italy eating fresh lemons is still believed, by many, to combat major epidemic infections. They are certainly very rich in minerals and vitamins, including B_1, B_2, B_3, carotene (pro-vitamin A), and C (up to 50mg per 100g of fruit).

Lemons remain popular in folk medicine as a remedy for feverish chills and coughs and numerous over-the-counter products based on honey and lemon mixtures are widely available. The essential oil is prepared from the peel so can often be heavily contaminated with pesticides unless produced from organically grown fruit. The oil is around 70% limonene and other constituents include pinene, myracene, citral, linalol, geraniol and citronellal.

Lemon oil diluted in water (or warm lemon juice) makes a good gargle for sore throats or diluted in sunflower oil can be used to relieve insect stings and the pain of neuralgia. Fresh lemon juice or slices of lemon make an acceptable alternative in both cases. Externally lemon juice can also be used to ease sunburn and irritant skin rashes. As a styptic it can be used on cotton wool swabs to speed clotting in nosebleeds and it will make an emergency antiseptic wash for cuts and grazes.

It is cleansing and stimulating and can also be useful added to rubs for arthritis, and rheumatism, especially where poor circulation is a factor or where there may be an infective cause.

Lemon is also popular in traditional beauty treatments to whiten the skin, the teeth, and encourage freckles to fade. Mixed with equal amounts of glycerine and eau de Cologne lemon juice makes a soothing and softening hand lotion.

Marjoram

Botanical name: *Origanum majorana*

Actions: analgesic, anaphrodisiac, antioxidant, antiseptic, antispasmodic, anti-viral, anti-bacterial, antifungal carminative, diaphoretic, digestive tonic, diuretic, emmenagogue, expectorant, hypotensive, laxative, nervine, sedative, peripheral vasodilator, wound herb

Extraction: by steam distillation of the dried flowering herb

Sweet marjoram is, like its close relative oregano (*O. vulgare*), most familiar as a culinary herb. "Oregano" reputedly derives from a Greek word meaning 'joy of the mountains', reflecting the plant's fortifying and uplifting effect. It has mainly been used in herbal medicine as a digestive remedy which is also soothing for menstrual problems and nervous tension. Writing in 1653, Nicholas Culpeper describes it as 'comforting in cold diseases of the head. . . the obstructions of the liver and spleen'.

The oil is warming for both mind and body and is similarly used for indigestion, constipation, period pains, pre-menstrual syndrome, nervous upsets and headaches but it is very effective for muscular aches and pains, sprains, strains, stiff joints and bruises. It can also ease lumbago and arthritis.

Caution: avoid the oil in pregnancy

Peppermint

Botanical name: *Mentha X piperita*

Actions: anti-spasmodic, digestive tonic, anti-emetic, carminative, peripheral vasodilator, diaphoretic, bile stimulant, analgesic

Extraction: by steam distillation of the flowering herb

Peppermint is a cross between spearmint and water mint and its characteristic smell is due to a high menthol content. Numerous varieties have been grown over the years; perhaps the most famous was Mitcham mint, a black peppermint which once formed an important cash crop in what are now London's southern suburbs.

The herb is largely used to relieve wind, bloating and colic, although it is also useful for catarrh and travel sickness.

The oil is used in creams and lotions for skin problems, and in steam inhalants for catarrh, sinusitis and head colds. It is also helpful for asthma, bronchitis and digestive upsets.

It can be useful in combinations for muscle pain and neuralgia, and is also stimulating to combat feelings of faintness, mental fatigue and nervous stress.

Caution: do not use peppermint with children under the age of four as the menthol content can be irritant for mucous membranes

Pine

Botanical name: *Pinus* spp.

Actions: anti-microbial, analgesic, anti-rheumatic, antiseptic, anti-viral, cholagogue, diuretic, expectorant, hypertensive, stimulant, vermifuge. Topically: rubefacient, insecticidal

Extraction: by dry distillation of the needles (*P. sylvestris*) or by steam distillation of sawdust and wood chippings (*P. palustris*)

Both Scots pine (*P. sylvestris*) and long-leaf pine (*P. palustris*) are used in aromatherapy. Scots pine is rather more common and as an effective antiseptic cough remedy is included in many decongestant and expectorant mixtures—such as throat lozenges and syrups—for coughs and colds. Pine oil is largely (up to 90%) made up of monoterpenes including pinene, limonene and camphene as well as bornyl acetate and citral.

It is a stimulating nervine and is used in aromatherapy for nervous exhaustion, stress-related problems and fatigue. It makes a useful addition to steam inhalations for colds and catarrh and the oil is also added to rubs for urinary infections and cystitis.

The oil is topically rubefacient so is used in a variety of external rubs for muscle stiffness and rheumatism, arthritis, gout and general muscular pains. Pine oil is a popular ingredient in many relaxing bath products targeted at backache sufferers.

Long-leaved pine is quite different chemically, and its constituents include terpineol, fenchyl alcohol and borneol. It has a more limited range of applications and is mainly used for respiratory problems and muscular aches and pains. It can help to ease lumbago, arthritis, sciatic pains, rheumatic aches and general muscle stiffness.

Both oils are equally useful for treating joint pains although Scots pine has a wider range of applications.

Caution: avoid in allergic skin conditions

Rosemary
Botanical name: *Rosmarinus officinalis*
Actions: leaves—antiseptic, anti-depressive, anti-spasmodic, astringent, cardiac tonic, carminative, cholagogue, circulatory stimulant, diaphoretic, digestive remedy, diuretic, nervine, restorative tonic for nervous system. Essential oil (topically) analgesic, anti-rheumatic, rubefacient
Extraction: by steam distillation of the fresh flowering tops

Rosemary is traditionally associated with remembrance—sprigs were exchanged by lovers or scattered on coffins. It is an apt association as rosemary has a stimulating effect on the nervous system and a reputation for improving the memory. The plant originates from the Mediterranean area and was first grown in Britain in the 14th century. It was regarded as uplifting and energising; or as Gerard said, 'it comforteth the harte and maketh it merie'.

As a nerve tonic it can be helpful for temporary fatigue and overwork. It makes a pleasant tea and will also stimulate the circulation and can relieve headaches, migraines, indigestion, and the cold feeling that comes with poor circulation. Since rosemary is an evergreen, the tea can be made using fresh herb throughout the year.

The oil contains pinenes, camphene, limonene, cineol and borneol—which is particularly stimulating for the nervous system and is also a valuable remedy for arthritis, rheumatism and muscular aches and pains.

Rosemary is reputed to darken greying hair, makes a good rinse for auburn, and will also help to clear dandruff.

Thyme
Botanical name: *Thymus vulgaris*
Actions: antibiotic, antiseptic, anti-spasmodic, anti-microbial, antitussive, astringent, carminative, diuretic, expectorant, wound herb. Topically: rubefacient
Extraction: by steam distillation from the fresh or partially dried flowering tops: 'red thyme' oil is the crude distillate which can be further distilled to produce 'white thyme' oil

Like many culinary herbs thyme is a soothing digestive remedy which can stimulate the digestion as it copes with rich foods. It is a useful expectorant, while the highly antiseptic oil makes it ideal both to clear phlegm and combat chest infections.

Common or garden thyme (*T. vulgaris*) is the cultivated form of wild thyme, *T. serpyllum*, which is known as 'mother of thyme'—possibly because of its traditional use for menstrual disorders. Wild thyme's botanical name is based on its creeping or serpent-like growth pattern and Pliny—in true Doctrine of Signatures fashion—recommended it as an antidote for serpent bites and 'the poison of marine creatures'. The Romans also burned the plant in the belief that the fumes would repel scorpions and 'all such creatures'.

The oil is mainly made up of thymol and carvacrol which are toxic phenols and can irritate the mucous membranes or cause sensitisation if used to excess. Lemon thyme and 'linalol'-type thyme oils are often less irritant, while white thyme is frequently synthetically adulterated.

Thyme oil has a wide range of uses in aromatherapy: it can be added to treatments for skin problems like acne and eczema as well as combating infections and infestations including lice and scabies. As a potent respiratory antiseptic it is good in chest rubs for bronchitis and asthma and is useful in inhalants for sinus problems, catarrh and colds. It can be used in abdominal massage for cystitis and indigestion and also acts as a strengthening nervine for stress-related problems and tension so is an ideal additive for a relaxing bath.

It is effective for muscular aches, pains and stiffness, gout, sprains, sports injuries and arthritis.

Tea tree
Botanical name: *Melaleuca alternifolia*
Actions: antiseptic, anti-bacterial, anti-fungal, anti-viral, immune stimulant, anti-parasitic
Extraction: by steam or water distillation from the leaves and twigs

European interest in the Australian tea tree dates back to the 1920s when the strong anti-bacterial action of its oil was first investigated in France.

Extracts were used in traditional Aboriginal medicine and in the past few years a thriving tea tree industry has grown up which has led to a number of highly adulterated oils appearing on the market. True tea tree oil is one of the few which does not usually irritate mucous membranes and it can be used neat on the skin.

The oil is useful for almost any infectious condition and can be helpful for locally infected joints in viral forms of arthritis.

Wintergreen
Botanical name: *Gaultheria procumbens*
Actions: analgesic, anti-inflammatory, anti-rheumatic, anti-tussive, astringent, carminative, diuretic, emmenagogue, galactagogue, stimulant
Extraction: by steam distillation of the leaves which have been previously macerated in warm water

Wintergreen was for generations the household standby for all sorts of muscle and joint pains: everything from lumbago and sciatica to neuralgia and rheumatism would be treated with vigorous massage using wintergreen ointments and extracts.

The oil is around 98% methyl salicylate (see **birch oil**, page 116) which, like aspirin, is a very effective anti-inflammatory and analgesic remedy. True wintergreen oil is very rare today and synthetic methyl salicylate is almost always substituted. This is an irritant and toxic chemical, especially if used neat or to excess, and many suggest it should be avoided altogether.

However, herbalists will still prescribe low doses of wintergreen internally for rheumatic problems and it is effective externally if used well diluted. A warming compress can easily be made by adding five drops of methyl salicylate (or wintergreen oil) to 500ml of hot water. Mix well and use to soak a cotton or linen cloth which can then be applied to aching limbs and muscles.

CHAPTER 6

Choosing the Right Diet

While alternative practitioners have long associated dietary problems with joint pains, the orthodox medical world is also becoming more receptive to the idea.

A Norwegian study in 1991 (quoted in McTaggart, 1992) found that a test group of rheumatoid arthritis sufferers improved significantly when they were given a gluten-free vegan diet followed by a lacto-vegetarian diet. The RA sufferers recorded marked reduction in tender and swollen joints, pain and stiffness, while grip strength increased significantly. These benefits were still present a year after the study ended. The research prompted an editorial in *The Lancet* (1991) to conclude that '. . . every rheumatology department needs a dietitian if not a health farm'.

A gluten-free vegan diet removes several of the most common allergens: gluten (found in wheat, oats, rye, and barley) itself; meat, especially beef and pork; and milk and dairy products. In addition, clinical ecologists have cited tobacco smoke, pesticides, perfume, hairspray, house dusts, mites, moulds and intestinal candidiasis as potential allergic causes for rheumatoid arthritis.

Avoiding the Wrong Foods
With food intolerance and poor digestive function contributory causes of miscellaneous joint pains and some forms of arthritis it is hardly surprising that 'arthritis diets' are so widely promoted.

Most emphasise the need to avoid acid residues from food which could contribute to the build-up of urates or oxalates in joints, leading to inflammation and damage. Gout sufferers also need to avoid purine-containing foods (see Chapter 2) so by the time all these various restrictions have been introduced it is hardly surprising that the poor arthritic feels there are very few food items left to choose from.

Foods labelled as leading to acidic residues and those which arthritics are usually urged to avoid include:

- most sources of animal protein, including meat, offal, poultry, eggs, fish and shellfish;
- wholegrain cereals and pulses/legumes (such as beans, peas and lentils);
- most seeds and nuts;
- vegetables and fruits high in oxalic acid, such as spinach, strawberries and sorrel;
- most citrus fruits, although grapefruit is generally tolerated;
- tomatoes and some other members of the Solanaceae (nightshade) family which includes aubergine, sweet peppers (capsicum), cayenne, paprika, potatoes and tobacco. (According to Heimlich, 1991) 70% of arthritics—in a study of 5,000 patients—who avoid nightshades gain relief: and
- all refined carbohydrates especially white flour and white sugar and products containing them such as most cakes, biscuits and white bread.

In addition long-term use of salicylates from aspirin can occasionally enhance salicylate sensitivity and a list of high-salicylate foods may be added to the 'foods to avoid' list. High-salicylate foods include:

- virtually all fruits except bananas, mangoes, paw-paws, peeled pears and pomegranates which are low in salicylates;
- most common vegetables including broad and green beans, asparagus, beetroot, broccoli, carrots, chicory, cucumber, courgettes, vegetable marrow, mushrooms, olives, onions, parsnips, radishes, sweetcorn, turnips and watercress, leaving little more than Brussels sprouts, cabbage, celery, leeks, lentils, lettuce, peas, swedes and soy products to choose from;

- most culinary herbs and spices;
- most fruit juices, tea, coffee, peppermint tea, Coca-Cola and all alcoholic drinks except gin and vodka;
- many common nuts including almonds, brazil nuts, coconut, macadamia nuts, peanuts, pine nuts, pistachio nuts, sesame seeds, walnuts and water chestnuts.

Clearly exclusion diets on this scale become totally impossible to maintain and a pragmatic approach is vital. The problem can be worse for the elderly arthritic with only a basic pension, or indeed any sufferers on a tight budget, as so many of the cheap staples—such as white bread or potatoes—are on the 'best avoided' list.

The long list of foods which can cause acid residues or are better avoided may seem to imply at best a lacto-vegetarian regime—but this does not suit everyone. Many who do opt for a vegetarian lifestyle find themselves lacking in energy, easily tired and with a weakened immune system. American doctor Peter d'Adamo has come up with one possible explanation based on our blood groups. These, suggest d'Adamo, provide the key to genetic evolution with each blood type suggesting where our ancestors originated. From this d'Adamo predicts personality and likely health problems.

- Those with Group O blood he sees as descended dominantly from the original prehistoric hunters, simple relaxed meat eaters with a strong constitution and plenty of physical energy.
- Group A individuals, he claims, are descended from the early farmers—capable of complex planning and working together but tending to be more preoccupied with detail so more likely to have problems relaxing and with a tendency to worry.
- Those with Group B blood, suggests Dr d'Adamo, originated in central Asia with the nomadic Mongol tribes, and people with this blood group tend to be flexible, creative and well balanced.
- Finally, he argues that Group AB is an amalgam of these

successive waves of European migration and d'Adamo sees these as a 'modern enigma', a confusing blend of the easy-going hunter, neurotic grain farmer and relaxed nomad.

Based on experience from both his father's and his own medical practices, Peter d'Adamo believes that Group Os are most likely to suffer from inflammatory diseases, including joint disorders, and allergies; the Group As will be most prone to heart disorders and cancer. Group B blood groups will be most liable to auto-immune disorders (such as psoriasis and RA) and chronic fatigue syndrome, while the ABs suffer the worst of all worlds with a high incidence of cancer and heart disease.

Much of his work is dismissed as largely speculative by the orthodox, but it is yet another attempt to predict our likely strengths, weaknesses and potential energy levels. Some who have tried his dietary advice—matching their food intake to blood group and historic or evolutionary connections (Os eating plenty of meat, As concentrating on grains etc.)—have found the therapy extremely energising.

Opting for a vegetarian diet might ease the joint pains of a sufferer with blood group O, but the resulting lethargy, lack of energy and additional health problems may be too high a price to pay.

Taking a Practical Approach

Avoiding excessive amounts of acidic foods and over-refined carbohydrate products is sensible advice for most people: many of us eat far more meat, fish and animal proteins than we actually need and a couple of vegetarian-only days each week is sensible advice for everyone.

If food intolerance is suspected, such as when the problem is very long-standing, possibly starting in childhood, where the digestive system is clearly also affected, or where there are recurrent infections due to the stresses of additional allergens on the immune system, then it can be worth trying an exclusion diet to pinpoint possible problems.

This is best undertaken in consultation with a health care

professional, which is especially important for the chronically or long-term ill.

In an exclusion diet each suspect food needs to be avoided completely for up to three weeks. If there is rapid weight loss in the first week (up to 2.3kg/5lb) together with an improvement in symptoms then it is very likely that this is the food that is causing problems. Similarly, the symptoms may appear to worsen for three or four days after the food is removed from the diet.

If none of this happens then reintroduce the food and see if there is any change in symptoms. Sometimes the improvement is so gradual that sufferers do not really believe that the test food was to blame and it is only when it is reintroduced and there is an acute flaring of symptoms that it is identified.

These challenges need to be repeated up to three times to be sure of identifying culprit foods, returning to a normal helping of the suspected food for seven to 10 days in between each challenge.

Groups of related food need to be eliminated together and likely culprits include:

- dairy products—cow's milk and milk products, goat's milk and milk products, butter, most margarine (except non-dairy products), all soya milk products, products containing milk, such as milk chocolate, biscuits and many convenience foods;
- meat—usual culprits may be beef, pork, bacon, sausages, preserved meats and chicken; generally tolerated are lamb, rabbit and game. Remember to avoid meat stocks, meat stock cubes, many soups, eggs and lecithin products;
- Solanaceae (nightshade) family—potatoes, aubergines, tomatoes, peppers (capsicum, cayenne, chillies, pimentos, paprika);
- gluten—gluten-containing cereals are wheat, oats, barley, and rye. Usually tolerated are rice, sago, tapioca, millet and buckwheat;
- corn (maize)—all products derived from corn including sweetcorn, corn oil, blended vegetable oils, baking powder, cornflour, corn syrup, cornflakes, custard powder,

many margarines, polenta, tortillas, popcorn and foods containing corn extracts (including some baked beans);
- salicylates (see above)—avoid all except the low-salicylate foods.

As well as identifying any possible food allergens contributing to the problem the diet should be as healthy as possible to encourage digestive function: plenty of fresh vegetables to provide fibre, meat and fish meals limited to no more than five days each week, a minimum of caffeine-containing drinks (i.e. tea, coffee and Coca-Cola limited to two cups per day), with at least two pints of spring or filtered water drunk each day instead.

Specific recommendations include:

Gout—avoid purine-containing foods (red meat, game, offal/organ meats, meat stock, fish, fish roes, shellfish, wholegrains, asparagus, cauliflower, mushrooms, spinach, pulses/beans and peas); avoid also alcohol (especially beer and sweet wines), excess fruit as fructose (fruit sugar) increases urate production, yeast-based flavourings, refined carbohydrates and saturated fats. Drink more fluids and eat high-fibre foods and green leafy vegetables as their folic acid content helps to reduce uric acid levels. Eat also plenty of celery, parsley and watercress and foods that are rich in zinc, magnesium and vitamin C (which also helps to increase uric levels in urine).

Osteoarthritis—as the weight-bearing joints (knees and hips) are commonly affected it makes sense to lose weight if necessary. Avoid refined carbohydrates and saturated fats which will also help to cut any excess weight. Avoid members of the Solanceae family, if they make symptoms worse: substitute more rice, buckwheat crêpes and pasta for potatoes as staple foods. Limit foods like tea, coffee and bran which can interfere with mineral absorption. Although bread made from brown flour is generally preferable to over-refined white bread, coarse wholemeal flour can have a similar effect on mineral absorption to bran so choose the finer brown bread options.

Rheumatoid arthritis — eat less acid-producing foods (basically most animal proteins, wholegrains, pulses and nuts) and eat more oily fish (see Chapter 7), fresh fruits and vegetables (especially green, leafy vegetables). Some sufferers find that a diet based on fish, brown rice, leafy vegetables and fruit can be helpful. Anti-inflammatory culinary herbs are also worth using: for example, ginger is a natural anti-inflammatory so adding a little freshly chopped root to stir fries and other dishes can help.

Rheumatism — eat more foods rich in zinc (including eggs, fish, meat, carrots, turnips, potatoes, garlic, seaweed, sprouted seeds, and nuts) as this mineral can help ease muscle pains, eat more fresh fruits and vegetables generally—especially celery and asparagus, which will help with diuresis, and cut down on alcohol; avoid caffeine-containing drinks, and cut sugar intake.

Cleansing Dishes

Many herbs can help to detoxify the system and reduce inflammation. By using them in cooking they can enhance the therapeutic effects of more conventional medication. Some herbs used for treating joint pains (see Chapter 4) can be added in cookery: angelica stems can be used as a flavouring for sweet and savoury dishes, seaweeds (like bladderwrack) are often included in oriental dishes, turmeric is ideal for flavouring spicy dishes, celery can be used in many soups and stews, while stinging nettles make an ideal cleansing soup. Others worth using regularly are coriander and ginger.

Coriander

Best known from its use in Indian and Middle Eastern cookery, coriander has become a familiar culinary herb over the past few years with a characteristic earthy flavour. Coriander seeds are a valuable medicinal herb traditionally used for minor digestive problems.

According to recent Japanese research coriander leaves can

140

accelerate the excretion of toxic metals such as mercury, lead and aluminium from the body. Unless they are removed by chemicals called 'chelating agents' these heavy metals remain in the body for ever, with high levels now blamed for certain arthritic conditions, depression, memory loss, muscle pain and weakness. Eating plenty of coriander is an inexpensive and easy way to remove (or 'chelate') toxic metals from the nervous system and body tissue. It can be added raw to soups or salad or used as a garnish with practically any dish.

Ginger
Ginger is both anti-inflammatory and is traditionally regarded in Chinese medicine as a detoxificant, often used with potentially dangerous herbs to modify their action. It also helps stimulate the digestion to cleanse the system so is ideal for inflammatory joint disorders associated with poor elimination of toxins.

Fresh coriander leaf pesto with pasta
Serves 4

1 handful fresh, organically grown coriander leaves, washed	2 tablespoons almonds, cashews, pine nuts
6 tablespoons olive oil	2 tablespoons lemon juice
1 clove of garlic	55g/2oz crumbled fetta cheese
	225g/8oz fresh pasta, such as spaghetti or tagliatelle

Garnish: Grated Parmesan cheese and freshly ground black pepper

Put the coriander and olive oil in food blender and process until finely chopped. Add the rest of the ingredients apart from the fetta cheese and process to a lumpy paste. The consistency can easily be changed by varying the amount of olive oil and lemon juice, but keep the 3:1 ratio of oil to juice. The pesto freezes well, so make several batches at once during the coriander season and store in small containers.

Cook the pasta as directed on the pack, drain well and spoon over the pesto immediately so that it melts into the hot pasta. Add the fetta cheese, toss well and sprinkle generously with grated Parmesan and freshly ground black pepper. Serve immediately.

Carrot–ginger soufflé with coriander sauce
Serves 4

1kg/1lb carrots
10g/½ oz butter
2–3 tablespoons water
200ml/8fl oz vegetable or chicken stock
25g/1oz fresh ginger, peeled and grated

2 cloves of garlic, crushed
2 eggs
½ teaspoon salt
½ teaspoon freshly ground black pepper

Sauce:

1 bunch of fresh coriander, washed, dried and finely chopped
1 garlic clove, crushed
1–2 tablespoons lime juice

3 tablespoons olive oil
½ teaspoon salt
½ teaspoon freshly ground black pepper

Heat the oven to 170°C/325°F/gas mark 3.

First make the soufflé: peel the carrots and cut a few of them lengthwise into thin bands. Cook the bands in the butter and water until they become soft and then line the sides of the four buttered, ovenproof ramekin dishes with the carrot bands. Slice the remaining carrots and boil them in the vegetable or chicken stock together with the grated ginger and garlic for 10–15 minutes. Drain well in a colander.

Blend the vegetables and egg well and season with salt and pepper to taste. Divide the mousse between the four ramekin dishes and bake in the preheated oven for about 20 minutes.

Meanwhile, make the sauce by combining the chopped coriander, crushed garlic, lime juice and oil in a bowl. Blend well and season with salt and pepper. When they are cooked, spoon a little of the sauce over the carrot soufflés and serve on their own as a starter or with a green salad for a light lunch.

Roast salmon with coriander pesto
Serves 4

5 garlic cloves, peeled but left whole

3 tablespoons extra virgin olive oil

4 pieces of salmon fillet with skin still attached: ideally use thick square pieces rather than long thin ones

seasoned flour

3–4 tablespoons coriander pesto (see above)

fresh basil or coriander leaves, shredded

Heat the oven to 200°C/400°F/gas mark 6.

Put the whole garlic cloves into a roasting dish with the olive oil and heat in the preheated oven for 15 minutes. Coat the salmon fillets in seasoned flour. Transfer the roasting dish to the hob and cook the salmon, skin side down, for two minutes.

Turn the oven up to 275°C/475°F/gas mark 9. Turn the salmon fillets skin side up and return the dish to the oven for three minutes. Serve the fillets on individual serving plates with mashed potatoes and a spoonful of the pesto. Garnish with the fresh herb leaves.

Stinging nettle soup
Serves 4

Nettle soup should really only be made in the spring as later in the year the nettles become coarse, unpleasant to eat—and they sting.

225g/8oz young nettle leaves

1l/1¾pt vegetable stock

1 medium-sized onion, chopped

1 medium-sized potato, chopped into small pieces

1 tablespoon olive oil

salt and freshly ground black pepper

crème fraîche

Remember to wear rubber gloves when preparing your nettles: wash and finely chop them. Heat the oil in a saucepan and sauté the onion and potato for two to three minutes, then add the vegetable stock and bring to a boil. Simmer for 10–15 minutes until the potato is soft and the stock is thickening. Add the chopped nettles and return to simmer for 10 minutes.

Season with salt and pepper to taste.

Serve with a spoonful of crème fraîche added to each bowl. If you prefer a smoother soup, blend with an electric food whisk or food processor and then reheat gently for one to two minutes before serving with the crème fraîche.

Fennel and celery soup
Serves 4

15g/½ oz butter
2 onions, chopped
1 fennel bulb, finely sliced
3 stalks of celery, finely sliced
1l/1¾ pt of chicken or vegetable stock
2 tablespoons soured cream

110g/4oz smoked ham or cooked bacon, cut into fine strips (optional)
salt and pepper to taste
1-2 tablespoons chopped fresh dill

Melt the butter in a large saucepan and sauté the chopped onions, fennel and celery for four to five minutes. Add the stock and simmer for about 15–20 minutes. Add the soured cream and reheat the soup taking care that it does not boil and curdle. Add the ham or bacon strips. Adjust seasonings (salt and pepper) to taste.

Serve sprinkled with a little chopped dill.

CHAPTER 7

Food Supplements and Additives

Many food supplements are recommended for joint pain sufferers: some can replace dietary imbalances related to the problem, others may strengthen the system to combat inflammation and bone degeneration. Typical regimes are reviewed first, followed by an overview of the various supplements involved.

Commonly Suggested Supplements

Backache: additional supplements are rarely appropriate for mechanical problems but manganese may be low in chronic sufferers and vitamin C (up to 5g daily) may help in some cases. Other common suggestions include: vitamins B, C, E, niacin, calcium, evening primrose oil.

Gout: supplements like vitamin C (up to 4g daily) can increase uric acid excretion; others can help restore normal digestion and metabolic function and suggestions include zinc (50mg daily), magnesium (300mg), bromelain (200mg), folic acid (30mg), vitamin C (3g), vitamin E (200iu), iron and magnesium.

Muscle pains: supplements can help with metabolic function to clear toxins—common suggestions include vitamin B_6, B_{12}, niacin, magnesium, calcium, zinc.

Osteoarthritis: supplements are mainly aimed at reducing inflammation and improving any associated mineral deficiencies and can include evening primrose oil or starflower oil, fish oils, iron, copper, zinc (25mg), selenium, manganese, vitamins A (*beta*-carotene up to 7,500iu), B (especially nicotinamide up to 1–4g per day; B_5, 10mg daily; or B_6, 25mg daily), C, and E (400iu daily). Extracts of green-lipped mussels and organic silicon also have their supporters.

Rheumatoid arthritis: supplements are mainly aimed at reducing inflammation while some argue that high levels of zinc can combat infecting agents contributing to the problem. Zinc (30–40mg daily), copper, manganese, vitamins B_6, B_3, B_5 (50mg) and C (up to 3g daily), nicotinamide (1–4g daily), evening primrose oil (up to 2,000mg daily), fish oils, tryptophan, histidine, and bromelain (250 mg).

Tenesynovitis, bursitis, fibrositis: injections of vitamin B_{12} have been recommended (Davies and Stewart, 1987). Others suggest vitamin B_6, calcium and magnesium (Bartram, 1995).

Essential Fatty Acids

Fatty acids are the building blocks for fats in the human body and are major components of cell membranes so play an important role in building and maintaining healthy cells. These acids are classified by molecular structure based on the number of carbon atoms they contain and the shape of the carbon chain. They are grouped as:

- ω (omega)3—which includes *alpha*-linolenic acid, stearidonic acid, eicosapentaenoic acid, docasahexaeoic acid;
- ω 6—including linoleic acid, *gamma*-linolenic acid, and arachidonic acid;
- ω 9 or monounsaturated acids—including oleic acid which is found in olive oil; and
- saturated fatty acids such as butyric acid found in butter.

Saturated acids are burned in the body to provide energy while the other unsaturated acids are of varying importance in body metabolism.

The most important fatty acids are the essential fatty acids:

- linoleic acid (*cis*-ω6,9-octadecadienoic acid); and
- linolenic acid (*cis*-ω3,6,9-octadecatrienoic acid).

The human body cannot metabolise these acids, although they form the basis of a number of important acids which it can make, so any shortfall in dietary intake of these chemicals leads to ill health.

Typical deficiency symptoms of linoleic acid include eczema, hair loss, liver and kidney degeneration, behavioural disturbances, recurrent infections, sterility, arthritis, circulatory problems and growth retardation. Typical deficiency symptoms of linolenic acid include general weakness, growth problems, visual impairment, learning difficulties and behavioural changes. Clearly these chemicals are vital for good health (Erasmus, 1986).

Both acids are found in plants with the richest sources being seed and nut oils, especially linseed, pumpkin and walnut oils.

Several vital fatty acids are needed by the body but can be made from either linoleic or linolenic acid. These include: *gamma*-linolenic acid (GLA), arachidonic acid, stearidonic acid, eicosapentataenoic acid (EPA) and docasahexaenoic acid (DHA). However, any failure of the necessary metabolic pathway can result in deficiency of these chemicals and this can cause a range of degenerative disorders including joint deterioration and skin problems.

The metabolic pathway for making these important acids is also quite complex and slow, so many argue that supplements which are rich in these chemicals can be beneficial. Equally, because dietary intake of linolenic acid tends to be low (it is only found in a few substances and many people never eat these) then supplements of the acid it makes can be helpful even if there is no problem with body metabolism.

Gamma-linolenic acid (GLA)

GLA is a precursor of prostaglandins E_1 which inhibits abnormal cell proliferation. During the 1970s researchers identified that the seeds of evening primrose oil were a rich source of GLA and since then the plant has been widely cultivated and its oil extensively marketed.

A healthy metabolism can produce GLA from linoleic acid, which is more commonplace than naturally occurring linolenic acid and is found in high concentration in walnut, safflower, sunflower and grape oils as well as in most nuts. The metabolic pathway for its production can be affected by poor diet and high cholesterol levels. As well as combating degenerative disorders and rheumatic problems, GLA is also reputed to ease menstrual and menopausal problems, strengthen the circulatory system and boost the immune system. Numerous studies (see Erasmus, 1986) over the years have confirmed GLA's efficacy and it is available in the UK as a prescription remedy for eczema and mastalgia (breast pains).

Naturally occurring evening primrose oils seeds usually average around 9% of GLA, while new strains and extraction techniques now produce levels of up to 25%. As well as evening primrose, GLA is found in borage and blackcurrant seeds and these are also available commercially with borage extracts usually marketed as starflower oil. Borage oil contains up to 24% GLA.

Recommendations on dosage vary: clinical trials have used dosages as high as 3–5g a day to treat irritable bowel syndrome associated with the menstrual cycle. Typically, the daily recommended dose of evening primrose or starflower oil will be around 500mg.

Eicosapentataeonic acid (EPA) and docasahexaenoic acid (DHA)
These ω3 acids are also essential for health and their lack has also been cited as a major cause of degenerative disorders including cancers and various forms of joint disease. EPA is the basis of prostaglandins E_3 series which can combat excess stickiness in blood platelets so help prevent blood clots which can contribute to heart attacks and strokes.

These acids are found in oily fish such as fresh salmon, sardines, mackerel, trout and eel, and many studies have pointed not only to a low incidence of heart problems but also fewer degenerative diseases—like arthritis—among populations eating a largely fish diet.

Clinical trials have also confirmed their efficacy: one 1985 double-blind study (quoted in McTaggart, 1992) found that 20 arthritis patients gained relief from taking 15 capsules a day of maxEPA (the equivalent of a single portion of fatty fish like salmon). However, excess fish oil can lead to changes in white blood cell counts and excess bleeding in the brain, so eating much more than the equivalent of one helping of fish per day can be dangerous.

Another Swedish study (quoted in Hubbard, 1995) by L. Skoldtsam at Kalmar Hospital, concluded that 10g of fish oil a day was as effective as NSAIDs, while tests by C. S. Lau at Ninewells Hospital in Dundee, found that patients taking fish oil supplements could reduce their NSAID medication significantly without suffering any deterioration in condition.

Minerals
Numerous minerals are needed by the body for vital functions and again their deficiency can lead to health problems which may be associated with joint pains.

Calcium
Calcium is essential to maintain healthy bones and teeth and is also involved in a number of biochemical processes. Calcium is found in dairy products, leafy vegetables, pulses, nuts and seeds (especially sesame). Dietary deficiency is not usually a problem, but absorption can be affected by bran and a high-fat diet, both commonplace among the elderly. Calcium supplements in arthritic disorders are generally designed to combat this absorption deficiency problem.

Copper and copper bracelets
The average adult has around 60–110mg of copper in the body so only tiny amounts are needed but it is essential. Copper deficiency is associated with anaemia, bone defects, nervous

system degeneration, reproductive problems, raised blood cholesterol levels, immune system problems and disorders in skin pigmentation.

Copper is found in many vegetables although the content does vary depending on the metal content of the soil: oysters, kidney, dried pulses, liver and nuts are all reliable copper-rich foodstuffs.

Copper deficiency has been associated with a tendency towards arthritic disorders and many people find that wearing a copper bracelet gives relief from pain. The practice is generally dismissed as superstitious nonsense by orthodox practitioners; however, an Australian study by Dr Ray Walker (quoted in Davies and Stewart, 1987) found that the copper bracelets lost on average 13mg in weight each month suggesting that minute quantities were dissolved in sweat and might then be absorbed through the skin. In all, 31 of Dr Walker's trial group of 40 arthritic patients felt better when wearing the bracelet.

Copper deficiency is known to limit the production of the enzyme superoxide dismutase which 'mops up' toxins produced in the body which are associated with inflammation and pain. Copper also reacts with salicylates and phenylbutazone so may be acting as a more efficient distribution mechanism for the drugs, carrying them through the body.

Whatever the reason, wearing a copper bracelet seems to help many arthritis sufferers and can be a very simple means of easing pain.

Iron

Iron is essential for producing the haemoglobin of our red blood cells and is thus vital for oxygen transport around the body. Deficiency is common in menstruating women and can lead to iron-deficient anaemia. It is often included in multi-vitamin/multi-mineral supplements but excess can lead to constipation. Its use in arthritis is generally based on presumed deficiency and thus a need to boost the blood transport mechanism which may be contributing to poor elimination and tissue health.

Magnesium

Magnesium is important in cell mechanism as well as needed for bone and teeth formation. Average daily requirement is around 400–800mg and deficiency can be common if the diet is high is refined and heavily processed foods. As with calcium, bran can also reduce absorption. Magnesium supplements are often given for premenstrual problems.

Manganese

Around 12–20mg of manganese are found in the average healthy human and it is essential for the bones, soft tissues, pituitary gland, liver and kidneys in some little-understood way.

Manganese deficiency can lead to problems with spinal discs and cartilage, middle ear imbalance, birth defects, fertility problems, reduced brain function and glucose intolerance. The body loses around 4mg a day of manganese so only tiny amounts are needed. Leafy vegetables and whole grains are the main sources and tea is a good source—one cup contains about 1mg.

Supplements are often recommended for arthritis but no more than 4mg per day need be taken.

Selenium

Selenium, a rare metallic element, is a key component of seleno-proteins which are necessary for normal health. They include anti-oxidant glutathione peroxidase enzymes which remove hydrogen peroxide and both lipid and phospholipid hydroperoxides which are created in the system by free radicals and can damage cell tissues. Selenium is also essential for control of thyroid hormone and for normal reproductive function.

We obtain our selenium from plants which extract the chemical from the soil, and in those areas which are naturally deficient in selenium, deficiency diseases—notably heart problems and deforming type of arthritis—are commonplace.

In Britain selenium intake has fallen in recent years partly due to changes in food supply; North American wheat for bread-making, for example, is particularly rich in selenium but as supplies switch to European sources so this source of selenium has diminished. The bioavailability of selenium has also been affected by acid rain converting the naturally occurring mineral into less accessible salts. Excess use of artificial fertilisers has also reduced plant absorption of minerals from the soil (Anon, 1997).

Selenium deficiency seems commonplace (Davies and Stewart, 1987) in patients suffering from liver disease, cancer, cardiovascular disease and older arthritics for reasons that are not completely clear. It could be part of a more widespread deficiency issue or to do with inefficient mineral absorption due to an unknown cause. However, studies suggest that these patients do respond to selenium supplements although, as with manganese, only tiny amounts are needed and the toxic dose is 800µg/day. Typically supplements of 100–200µg/day are adequate (Hubbard, 1995) usually in the form of selenomethionine in brewer's yeast, sodium selenate, or selenium-enriched kelp. Brazil nuts are a good natural source.

Zinc
Zinc deficiency is associated with a wide range of disorders including slow growth, infertility, hair loss, immune deficiency, skin problems, diarrhoea and night blindness. Its shortage has also been linked with connective tissue disease.

Zinc is found in many foods especially muscle meats such as chops and steak, oysters, ginger, most nuts, egg yolk, oats, wholewheat, potatoes, garlic, carrots, turnips and beans, so a healthy diet should provide plenty. However, strict vegetarians may not obtain enough from their food nor may those on a limited income who eat fewer of the more expensive muscle meats. Absorption can also be affected by excess bran in the diet (popular with many elderly people who believe that it will combat constipation) or by taking iron tablets. Zinc loss is also accelerated by penicillamine drugs used in some treatments for arthritis.

Zinc is believed to help strengthen the immune system and is often combined with vitamin C as anti-infection supplements for the winter. It also affects prostate function and, again, is often included in products targeted at older men. Low levels of zinc have been reported in many rheumatoid arthritis sufferers and in trials, those given zinc supplements (Davies and Stewart, 1987) did report marked improvements in joint swelling, morning stiffness and joint tenderness.

Vitamins
Vitamins are dietary substances needed by the body in tiny amounts for normal biochemical function. They are generally divided into two groups: fat-soluble (A, D, E and K) and water soluble (B and C). They are widely used in supplements although a good diet high in fresh, organically grown produce should contain an adequate amount for the healthy.

Vitamin A
A number of fat-soluble compounds, including retinol, retinal and retinoic acid only found in animal produce (liver, kidney, whole-fat milk, butter and egg yolk) are loosely grouped as vitamin A. Some of these vitamin-A-type compounds are found in vegetables, generally as orange/yellow pigments, and these are water soluble. The most important is *beta*-carotene. Vitamin A is important for eye function; it prevents drying of the eye and corneal changes and is necessary for normal retinal function especially light-sensitive capabilities associated with night blindness.

Vitamin A is also important for maintaining the stability of cell membranes—hence recommended for arthritics where breakdown of the synovial membrane is a problem—and is believed to be helpful in pregnancy to prevent birth defects. Vitamin A can be toxic in excess.

Vitamin B complex
Vitamin B is a complex group of chemicals which are all water-soluble and found in such foods as brewer's yeast, meats, wholegrain cereals, and vegetable proteins. They are chemically distinct but interact within the body in a number of metabolic processes. Deficiency of individual B vitamins is rare, but occurs sometimes with vitamin B_{12}, which is generally only found in animal products so can be missing from strictly vegetarian diets. The B vitamins are referred to both by number and name, which can be confusing.

- Vitamin B_1 (thiamin)—important in energy production and carbohydrate mechanism.
- Vitamin B_2 (riboflavin)—needed for production of enzymes mainly found in the liver and important in oxidising compounds to produce energy.
- Vitamin B_3 (nicotinic acid, also known as niacin, and nicotinamide)—used in hydrogen transport and enzyme production. Nicotinic acid is important in cholesterol metabolism and high doses have been recommended for osteoarthritis, especially of the knees, although the evidence is largely anecdotal. Nicotinamide is often suggested as a supplement for arthritics.
- Vitamin B_5 (pantothenic acid)—regarded as a lesser B vitamin, B_5 is important in reactions involving carbohydrates, fats and amino acids.
- Vitamin B_6 (pyridoxine, pyridoxal and pyridoxamine)—important in protein metabolism and needed by the body in direct proportion to the amount of protein consumed. B_6 is also involved in the metabolism of essential body chemicals including histamine, hydroxytryptamine and serotonin, which is important in brain chemistry, so deficiency of vitamin B_6 can affect behaviour. Many women find vitamin B_6 supplements helpful for premenstrual problems, although recent health scares over the ill-effects of high doses have reduced the popularity of this approach.
- Vitamin B_{12} (cyanocobalamin)—important in cell formation and production of red blood corpuscles, a deficiency of B_{12} can lead to pernicious anaemia.
- Biotin—a lesser known B vitamin; deficiency is believed to contribute to severe cradle cap in babies and scaly dermatitis in adults.
- Choline—essential in human nutrition and fat metabolism, choline is related to other B vitamins and is a constituent of lecithin. It also forms acetyl-choline which is important in the transmission of nerve impulses. Supplements have been given for neurological diseases, including Alzheimer's.

- Folic acid—closely linked with B_{12}, folic acid is important for healthy function of the central nervous system and also in blood formation. Supplements in pregnancy are believed to reduce the risk of spina bifida.
- Inositol—like choline, this is involved in fat metabolism and levels are often high in diabetics and those with kidney disease. It may be involved in nerve disorders found in diabetics.

Vitamin C

Vitamin C helps to maintain healthy connective tissues and bones and is involved in the normal metabolism of cholesterol. Deficiency leads to scurvy, which was once common on long sea voyages, with bleeding and poor wound healing. Vitamin C is water-soluble and also involved in the protection of cortisol by the adrenal glands.

Vitamin C is a very widely used supplement and its supporters credit it with prevention of a range of ills from the common cold to cancer. It is an effective antioxidant and is also anti-viral and anti-bacterial. Dosages of up to 5g a day can be safely taken, although in high doses it can contribute to diarrhoea. Vitamin C is found in fresh fruits and vegetables but is destroyed in cooking and breaks down rapidly after harvesting so is highest in the freshest vegetables.

Dosages up to 3,000mg daily (Hubbard, 1995) have been recommended for arthritics although at this level side effects can be commonplace and it is better to maintain high doses for short periods only or use 500–1,000mg daily instead.

Vitamin E

Vitamin E is also known as tocopherol and is sometimes called the 'anti-old age' vitamin. The vitamin is fat-soluble and found in many vegetable oils, nuts, lettuce and eggs. It is an antioxidant and is believed to act as nature's preservative, helping prevent fats from going rancid. It can help protect the lungs from pollutants and is often given as a supplement to those with high blood pressure or heart problems.

Vitamin E can also reduce the risk of inflammation so can be helpful in inflammatory rheumatic disorders. Typical daily doses of 400iu are generally recommended for arthritis (Hubbard, 1995).

Assorted Food Supplements

New Zealand green-lipped mussels

Green-lipped mussels (*Perna canaliculus*) from New Zealand have been studied since the 1960s, at first as possible therapeutic agents for treating cancer. While the extracts had little effect on cancer, patients involved in trials reported an easing of rheumatic aches and pains when they were taking the extracts, and since then the mussels have been widely promoted as an arthritic remedy.

Green-lipped mussels filter up to 72 litres of ocean water daily as they extract the plankton and algae on which they feed; these are converted into various nutrients including mucopolysaccharides which are believed to be the active agent in easing joint stiffness and pain when the mussels or mussel extracts are then eaten by human arthritis sufferers.

Usual dose is initially around 1,000mg of mussel extract daily followed by a maintenance dose of around 250mg daily when symptoms ease.

Organic silicon

Organic silicon products are also regarded by some enthusiasts as an effective remedy for arthritic and rheumatic problems. Silicon is found in many of the strong tissues of the body (such as arterial walls, skin and cornea) and is also important for building cartilage and connective tissue in ways that are not fully understood. Silicon is found in plants like bamboo and horsetail as well as rye, millet, barley, potatoes and wholewheat, with traces found in artichokes, corn, asparagus, rice, sunflower seeds and parsley. Although these are important food sources they form only a small part of the modern diet and are often highly processed. In addition, silicon is notoriously difficult to extract during normal digestive processes—herbalists who use horsetail as a source of silicon need to simmer the plant for some hours before making extracts in order to ensure a high silicon content.

The result is likely to be silicon deficiency and some believe that this is a prime cause of arthritic problems as we grow older.

Organic silicon is obtained from micro-organisms in the soil which dissolve the silicon on the layer of sand grains and create a fine layer of amorphous silicon which is water-soluble and can be readily absorbed in normal digestion. Work on using organic silicon extracts for arthritis and rheumatism began in the 1950s, drawing on traditional North African practices of burying sufferers up to their necks in hot sand for 30 minutes every two weeks in order to obtain benefit from the organic silicon found naturally there.

Silica products are now readily available and many are designed for topical treatment (as in the North African model); others are for internal use and may combine organic silicon with anti-inflammatory herbs like meadowsweet.

Amino acids

Amino acids, the building blocks for the body's various proteins, are sometimes added to dietary supplements. The full complement is found in animal products but plant proteins usually contain only a selection, which is why vegetarians should eat both pulses and grains together in order to balance amino acid intake. The individual acids have a number of therapeutic uses including in rheumatoid arthritis, recurrent infections and fertility treatment. Amino acids used in food supplements include: arginine, cysteine, cystine, histidine, isoleucine, leucine, lysine, methionine, phylalanine, taurine, tryptophan, tyrosine and valine.

Bromelain

Bromelain is an enzyme found in fresh pineapple and is now extracted and marketed as a food supplement which can stimulate digestion. This protolytic enzyme is very similar to papain, found in papaya fruits which are traditionally eaten in the East for digestive problems.

Both enzymes have a local action on the digestive tract but are not significantly absorbed into the system, so they do not affect the liver. Both papain and bromelain are used in food supplements where they are generally suggested for indigestion and gastritis, although they can also be a useful part of a cleansing routine aimed at stimulating the digestion to improve elimination and clear toxins.

Some commercial products combine papaya and pineapple extracts together.

References and Further Reading

Anon (1997) *British Medical Journal*, **314**, 387–8, quoted in *Greenfiles*, 11(2), 21–2.

Bartram, T. (1995) *Encyclopedia of Herbal Medicine*, Grace Publishers, Christchurch.

Beatty, C. (1999) 'The use of filipendula and prescribing for arthritis by medical herbalists', *The European Journal of Herbal Medicine*, **5**(1), 26–8.

Belaiche, P. (1982) 'Étude clinique du 630 cas d'arthrose traités par le nébulisat aquex d'*Harpagophytum procumbens* (radix)', *Phytotherapy*, **1**, 22–8.

Beinfield, H., and Korngold, E. (1991) *Between Heaven and Earth: A Guide to Chinese Medicine*, Ballantine Books, New York.

Bone, K. (1991) 'Turmeric—the spice of life?' *British Journal of Phytotherapy*, **2**(2), 51–60.

Bown, D. (1995) *Encyclopaedia of Herbs and their Uses*, Dorling Kindersley, London.

Brooks, P. M., and Day, R. O. (1991) *New England Journal of Medicine*, 13 June 1991, quoted in McTaggart, L. (1992) *op. cit.*

Carle, R. (1990) Anti-inflammatory and spasmolytic botanical drugs, *British Journal of Phytotherapy*, **1**, 33–9.

Chevallier, A. (1996) *Encyclopaedia of Medicinal Plants*, Dorling Kindersley, London.

Chopra, A., *et al.* (2000) 'Randomized double blind trial of an Ayurvedic plant-derived formulation for the treatment of rheumatoid arthritis', *Journal of Rheumatology*, **27**(6), 1365–72.

Chrubasik, S., Zimpfer, C., Schutt, U., and Ziegler, R. (1996) 'Effectiveness of *Harpagophytum procumbens* in treatment of acute low back pain', *Phytomedicine*, **3**(1), 1–10.

Chrubasik, S., Enderlein, W., Bauer, R., and Grabner, W. (1997) 'Evidence for antirheumatic effectiveness of *Herba urtica dioicae* in acute arthritis: A pilot study', *Phytomedicine*, **4**(2), 105–8.

d'Adamo, P., and Whitney, C. (1998) *The Eat Right Diet*, Century, London.

Davies, S., and Stewart, A. (1987) *Nutritional Medicine*, Pan Books, London.

Deodhar, S. D., Sethi, R., and Srimal, R. C. (1980) 'Preliminary study of anti-rheumatic activity of curcumin', *Indian Journal of Medical Research*, **71**, 632–4.

Dombradi, C. A., and Foldeak, S. (1966) 'Anti-tumour activity of A. lappa extract', *Tumori*, **52**, 173–5.

Ebringer, A. (1991) *Bacterial antibodies in ankylosing spondylitis and rheumatoid arthritis*. Report to the Arthritis and Rheumatism Council.

Erasmus, U. (1986) *Fats and Oils*, Alive Books, Vancouver.

ESCOP (1997) *Monograph: Urtica folium*, European Scientific Co-operative on Phytotherapy, Exeter.

Foster, S. (1999) 'Black Cohosh: a literature review', *Herbalgram*, No. 45, pp. 35–45.

Franchomme, P. (1985) *Advanced therapy for infectious diseases*, International Phytomedical Foundation, France; Seminar on Germicidal Oils, 24–25 November 1985, London.

Franchomme, P., and Peoel, D. (1991) *L'Aromathérapie Exactement*, Jollais, Limoge.

Frawley, D., and Lad, V. (1986) *The Yoga of Herbs*, Lotus Press, Santa Fe.

Gattefossé, R.-M. (1937) *Aromathérapie*; English translation by R. Tisserand as *Gattefossé's Aromatherapy* (1993), C. W. Daniel, Saffron Walden.

Grennan, D. M. (1984) *Rheumatology*, Ballière Tindall, London.

Groenewegen, W. A., Knight, D. W., and Heptinstall, S. (1992) 'Progress in the medicinal chemistry of the herb feverfew', *Progress in Medicinal Chemistry*, **29**, 217–38.

Gursche, S. (1993) *Healing with Herbal Juices*, Alive Books, Vancouver.

Harrison, J. (1984) *Love Your Disease*, Angus & Robertson, Sydney.

Heimlich, J. (1991) *What Your Doctor Won't Tell You*, HarperPerennial, New York; study also reported in *J. Int. Acad. Prev. Med.*, November 1982.

Hobbs, C. (1995) *Medicinal Mushrooms*, Botanica Press, Santa Cruz.

Hoffman, D. (1983) *The Holistic Herbal*, Findhorn Press, p. 195.

Holmes, P. (1989) *The Energetics of Western Herbs*, Artemis Press, Boulder, Colorado.

Hubbard, B. (1995) 'Arthritis: second-line terrors', *What Doctors Don't Tell You*, **5**(5), 1–3.

Lecomte, A., and Costa, J. P. (1992) 'Harpagophytum dans l'arthrose; Étude en double insu contre placebo', *37°2 Le Magazine*, **15**, 27–30.

Leirisalo-Repo, M., *et al.* (1997) *Ann. Rheum. Dis.*, **56**(9), 516–20.

McTaggart, L. (1992). 'Arthritis: the price of painkillers', *What Doctors Don't Tell You*, **2**(12), 1–3.

Matthews, R. (2000) 'Breakthrough as scientists discover cure for arthritis.' *Sunday Telegraph*, 29 October, 2000, p. 1. Preview of study presented to the American College of Rheumatology, 30 October 2000, and to be published in *Rheumatology*.

McIntyre, A. (1996) *The Complete Floral Healer*, Gaia Books, London.

Mehra, K. S., Mikuni, I., Gupta, V., and Gode, K. D. (1984) '*Curcuma longa* drops in coreal wound healing', *Tokai Journal of Experimental and Clinical Medicine*, **9**, 27–31.

Mills, S. Y., *et al.* (1996) *Br. J. Rheumatology*, **35**, 784–878.

Newall, C. A., Anderson, L. A., and Phillipson, J. D. (1996) *Herbal Medicines: a guide for health care professionals*, The Pharmaceutical Press, London.

Ody, P. (1997) *100 Great Natural Remedies*, Kyle Cathie, London.

Ody, P. (2000) *The Complete Guide: Medicinal Herbal*, Dorling Kindersley, London.

Ody, P., Lyon, A., and Vilinac, D. (2000) *The Chinese Herbal Cookbook*, Kyle Cathie, London.

Page, J., and Henry, D. (2000) *Arch. Intern. Med.*, **160**(6), 777–84.

Pinget, M., and Lecomte, A. (1988) '*The effects of Harpagophytum arkocelules in degenerative rheumatology*', Arkopharma research paper.

Ramm, S., and Hansen, C. (1995) 'Brennessel-Extrakt bei rheumatischen Beschwerden', *Deutsch. Apoth Ztg*, **135**(suppl), 3–8.

Ramm, S., and Hansen, C. (1996) 'Brennessbläter-extrakt bei arthrose und rheumatoider arthritis', *Therapiewoche*, **28**, 3–6.

Randall, C., *et al.* (1999) *Complementary Therapeutics and Medicine*, **7**(3), 126–31.

Rovesti, P., and Gattefossé, H. M. (1973) *Labo-Pharma. Probl. Techn*, **223**, 32–8.

Srimal, R. C., Khana, N. M., and Dhawan, B. N. (1971) 'A preliminary report on anti-inflammatory activity of curcumin', *Indian Journal of Pharmacology*, **3**, 10.

Srimal, R. C., and Dhawan, B. N. (1973) 'Pharmacology of diferuloyl methane (curcumin) a non-steroidal anti-inflammatory agent', *Journal of Pharmacy and Pharmacology*, **25**, 447–52.

Strehlow, W., and Hertzka, G. (1988) *Hildegard of Bingen's Medicine*, Bear & Co, Santa Fe, New Mexico.

Swiatek, L., *et al.* (1986) 'Content of phenolic acids in leaves of *Menyanthes trifoliata*', *Planta Med.*, **52**, 530.

Teeguarden, R. (1985) *Chinese Tonic Herbs*, Japan Publications, New York.

The Lancet (1991) editorial, *The Lancet*, 12 October 1991.

Tisserand, R. (1977) *The Art of Aromatherapy*, C. W. Daniels, Saffron Walden.

Veal, L. (1998) 'Wielding the birch', *Int. J. Alt. Comp. Med.*, May 1998, 17–19.

Viaud, H. (1983) *Huiles Essentielles, Hydrolats*, Editions Presence, Sisteron.

Weiss, R. F. (1988) *Herbal Medicine* (translated from the sixth edition of *Lehrbuch der Phytotherapie* by A. R. Meuss), Beaconsfield Publishers, Beaconsfield.

Wren, R. C. (1988) *Potter's New Cyclopaedia of Botanical Drugs and Preparations*, C. W. Daniels, Saffron Walden.

Yeung, H. C. (1988) *Handbook of Chinese Herbs and Formulas*, Institute of Chinese Medicine, Los Angeles.

Zeylstra, H. (1991) 'The phytotherapeutic approach to rheumatoid arthritis', *British Journal of Phytotherapy*, **2**(1), 15–20.

Zeylstra, H. (1998) '*Filipendula ulmaria*', *British Journal of Phytotherapy*, **5**(1), 8–12.

Glossary of Medicinal Terms

Adrenal cortex—part of the adrenal gland, located above the kidneys, which produces several steroidal hormones.

Alkaloid—active plant constituent containing nitrogen and which usually has a significant effect on bodily function.

Allergen—any substance which triggers an allergic response.

Analgesic—relieves pain.

Anaesthetic—causes local or general loss of sensation.

Anaphrodisiac—reduces sexual desire and excitement.

Anodyne—allays pain.

Antibiotic—destroys or inhibits the growth of micro-organisms.

Anti-bacterial—destroys or inhibits the growth of bacteria.

Anti-fungal—destroys or inhibits the growth of fungi.

Anti-inflammatory—reduces inflammation.

Anti-microbial—destroys or inhibits the growth of micro-organisms.

Antioxidant—prevents or slows the natural deterioration of cells due to oxidation that occurs as they age.

Anti-rheumatic—relieves the symptoms of rheumatism.

Antiseptic—controls or prevents infection.

Anti-spasmodic—reduces muscle spasm and tension.

Anti-tussive—inhibits the cough reflex, helping to stop coughing.

Aphrodisiac—promotes sexual excitement.

Arteriosclerosis—build-up of fatty deposits in the blood vessels leading to narrowing and hardening and associated with heart disease and strokes.

Astringent—used to describe a herb which will precipitate proteins from the surface of cells or membranes, thus producing a protective coating.

Bile—thick, bitter fluid secreted by the liver and stored in the gall bladder which aids the digestion of fats.

Bitter—stimulates secretion of digestive juices.

Blood clotting—the process by which the proteins in blood are changed from a liquid to a solid by an enzyme, in order to check bleeding.

Blood sugar—levels of glucose in the blood.

Bronchial—relating to the air passages of the lungs.

Bulk laxative—increases the volume of faeces producing larger, softer stools.

163

Capillary permeability—the exchange of carbon dioxide, oxygen, salts and water between the blood in capillaries and tissues.

Carcinogenic—causes cancer.

Carminative—relieves flatulence, digestive colic and gastric discomfort.

Cerebral circulation—blood supply to the brain.

Cholagogue—Stimulates bile flow from the gall bladder and bile ducts into the duodenum.

Cholesterol—fat-like material present in the blood and most tissues which is an important constituent of cell membranes, steroidal hormones and bile salts. Excess cholesterol has been blamed for the build-up of fatty deposits in the blood vessels seen in arteriosclerosis.

Circulatory stimulant—increases blood flow.

Citronellal—a volatile oil with a lemon aroma found in a number of herbs (including lemongrass) and used for flavourings and insect repellents.

Citronellol—a volatile oil with a rose-like aroma found in rose geranium and other species.

Cleansing herb—a herb that improves the excretion of waste products from the body.

Cooling—used to describe herbs that are often bitter or relaxing and will help to reduce internal heat and hyperactivity.

Coumarin—active plant constituent which affects blood clotting.

Decongestant—relieves congestion, usually nasal.

Demulcent—softens and soothes damaged or inflamed surfaces, such as the gastric mucous membranes.

Depressant—reduces nervous or functional activity.

Diaphoretic—increases sweating.

Diuretic—encourages urine flow.

Doctrine of Signatures—a mediaeval theory that plants gave a clue as to their properties in their appearance, for example yellow flowered plants were supposed to be good at treating jaundice because in jaundice the patient's skin appears yellow.

Emetic—causes vomiting.

Emollient—softens and soothes the skin.

Essential oil—volatile chemicals extracted from plants by such techniques as steam distillation; highly active and aromatic.

Expectorant—enhances the secretion or sputum from the respiratory tract so that it is easier to cough up.

Febrifuge—reduces fever.

Flavonoids—active plant constituents which improve the circulation and may also have diuretic, anti-inflammatory and anti-spasmodic effects.

Haemostatic—stops bleeding.

Hormone—a chemical substance produced in the body which can affect the way tissues behave. Hormones can control sexual function as well as emotional and physical activity.

GLOSSARY OF MEDICINAL TERMS

Hyperacidity—excessive digestive acid causing a burning sensation.

Hyperglycaemic—increases blood sugar levels.

Hypoglycaemic—reduces blood sugar levels.

Laxative—encourages bowel motions.

Lipids—fat-like chemicals (such as cholesterol) which are present in most tissues and are important structural materials for the body.

Menthol—a volatile oil with a peppermint aroma extracted from various mints (including peppermint) which is carminative, locally anaesthetic, decongestant and antiseptic. Used in a number of herbal products for colds and indigestion.

Mucilage—complex sugar molecules found in plants that are soft and slippery and provide protection for the mucous membranes and inflamed surfaces.

Nervine—herb that affects the nervous system and which may be stimulating or sedating.

Peripheral circulation—blood supply to the limbs, skin and muscles (including heart muscles).

Peristalsis—the waves of involuntary contractions in the digestive tract which move food and waste products through the system.

Phlegm—catarrhal-like secretion or sputum. In both Galenical and Oriental medicine phlegm is a more complex entity related in internal balance and sometimes associated with spleen deficiency.

Photosensitivity—sensitivity to light.

Physiomedicalism—system of medicine developed in 19th-century North America which focused on disease as a result of cold conditions.

Prostaglandins—hormone-like substances that have a wide range of functions in the body. They can act as chemical messengers and some also cause uterine contractions. Various series of prostaglandins are known usually designated PGE_1, PGE_2, etc.

Pungent—having an acrid smell and bitter flavour.

Purgative—drastic laxative.

Pyrrolizidine alkaloids—chemicals found in a number of plants (including comfrey, borage and coltsfoot) which in excess can be associated with liver damage although many regard the research evidence for this as inconclusive.

***Qi* (ch'i)**—the body's vital energy as defined in Chinese medicine.

Relaxant—relaxes tense and overactive nerves and tissues.

Rubefacient—a substance which stimulates blood flow to the skin causing local reddening.

Saponins—active plant constituents similar to soap and producing a lather with water. They can irritate the mucous membranes of the digestive tract which, by reflex, has an expectorant action. Some saponins are chemically similar to steroidal hormones.

165

Sedative—reduces anxiety and tension.

Simple—a herb used as a remedy on its own.

Soporific—induces drowsiness and sleep.

Stimulant—increases activity.

styptic—stops external bleeding.

Systemic—affecting the whole body.

Tannin—active plant constituents which are astringent and combine with proteins. The term is derived from plants used in tanning leather.

Thyroid—gland in the neck which controls metabolism and growth; it requires iodine for normal function.

Tonic—restoring, nourishing and supporting for the entire body.

Tonify—a tonic action: strengthening and restoring for the system.

Topical—local administration of a herbal remedy.

Warming—a remedy which increases body temperature and encourages digestive function and circulation. Warming herbs are often spicy and pungent to taste.

Yang—aspect of being equated with male energy—dry, hot, light, ascending.

Yin—aspect of being equated with female energy—damp, cold, dark, descending.

Consulting a
Medical Herbalist

While over-the-counter herbal remedies can be helpful for a range of ailments, more serious problems need professional help. Britain is probably unique within Europe in having a well-established and reputable system for training herbal practitioners who have not necessarily obtained any other medical qualifications.

The National Institute of Medical Herbalists was founded in 1864 and members qualify by examination after four or five years of specialist study. Many overseas students also attend courses run by the School of Phytotherapy in the UK in Sussex, and there are now two UK universities offering degree courses in herbal medicine. Members of the National Institute use the initials MNIMH or FNIMH after their names, which gives the patient some guarantee that they are consulting a suitably trained practitioner.

The UK's other main professional herbal body is The General Council and Register of Herbalists, whose members use the initials MH. It has a rather different philosophical approach from that usually adopted by the NIMH practitioners with its members tending more towards homoeopathy: herbal tinctures are likely to be prescribed in drop doses rather than the teaspoonful generally favoured by NIMH members. A third, more recently formed, organisation is the Register of Traditional Chinese Medicine whose members largely use a combination of acupuncture and Chinese herbs.

Consulting a professional herbalist is not all that different from visiting a GP—or rather, visiting a GP as one would have done 40 or 50 years ago. Indeed, many herbalists liken their approach to that of the old-fashioned family physician using a lot of patient listening and probing questions to uncover all the relevant symptoms along with time-honoured diagnostic techniques: feeling pulses, looking at tongues, testing urine; and with clinical examinations dependent on palpation, auscultation and percussion rather than laboratory tests. A first consultation will generally take at least an hour and subsequent ones 20 minutes or so.

As well as reviewing the current illness, the herbalist will ask about medical history: previous health problems that may be contributing to the current imbalance, family tendencies and allergies, diet, lifestyle, stresses and worries.

Examinations may include taking blood pressure and pulses, palpating the abdomen to identify the cause of pain or discomfort, listening to chest wheezes (auscultation) or checking the degree of movement in an arthritic knee or shoulder. Simple clinical tests undertaken on site could include urine analysis or measuring haemoglobin levels using a tiny drop of blood. Existing orthodox medication also needs to be checked.

Herbalists would certainly not recommend dropping vital drugs, but any incompatibility of these with herbal remedies obviously needs to be considered when prescribing plant medicines. Similarly, many patients turn to herbs because they are anxious to phase out their drugs, for whatever reason, and a safe programme of replacing them with gentler herbal remedies needs to be devised—preferably with the support and co-operation of the patient's GP. Herbal remedies, for example, can be very helpful for sufferers trying to break an addiction to tranquillisers or sleeping pills, or as alternatives for those suffering the side effects from NSAIDs used for arthritis.

At the end of the consultation, the patient does not simply leave with a prescription for the local pharmacist to dispense. In Britain, few pharmacies are willing to stock the hundreds of tinctures, creams, oils, powders, capsules or dried herbs that the medical herbalist needs to keep available, so all medical herbalists are permitted under the 1968 Medicines Act and The Medicines (Retail Sale and Supply of Herbal Remedies) Order 1977 to make and dispense their own remedies. As well as a combination of herbs, specially selected to help the unique health problems of each unique individual, the patient may leave the consultation room with a list of dietary suggestions, foods to avoid or details of those to eat more of. There may be recommended relaxation routines to follow or Bach Flower Remedies to help emotional factors affecting physical well-being. Or perhaps the patient will be sent away with a small growing plant to bring a little love and beauty into their life. Whatever the remedy, healing is a two-way process and the patient must take responsibility for their own health and actively participate in any cure. Those who expect a 'magic pill' to solve their problems, with little of their own effort, may be happier with orthodox therapies.

Generally herbalists like to see patients fairly soon after the first consultation to check on progress—perhaps after two or three weeks—with regular meetings every four to six weeks for six months or more in chronic cases. Herbal medication is likely to be altered slightly after each consultation to reflect changes in the condition.

Just as all patients are different so too are all herbalists. Finding a practitioner you can trust and with whom you feel empathy can be just as important in treatment as taking the right herbs. Some herbalists follow a semi-orthodox path prescribing remedies to ease symptoms just as modern drugs do; others will focus on holistic treatments urging major lifestyle changes. Some will only use Western herbs, others a combination of Chinese or Ayurvedic remedies. Some will talk mainly of pathological conditions, others will suggest *Qi* stagnation, allergies or define just about anything in terms of emotional stress. Some will depend on the consulting couch and the results of clinical tests for diagnosis; others will swing a pendulum or try kinesiology. If possible, choose your practitioner by personal recommendation from like-minded friends to ensure a good relationship with someone who understands your problem and whom you can also understand.

Suppliers and Contact Addresses

Associations and Professional Bodies
British Herbal Medicine Association, Sun House, Church Street, Stroud, Gloucestershire GL5 1JL.
The General Council and Register of Consultant Herbalists. Marlborough House, Swanpool, Falmouth, Cornwall TR11 4HW.
The Herb Society, Deddington Hill Farm, Warmington, Banbury, Oxon OX17 1XB.
National Institute of Medical Herbalists, 56 Longbrook Street, Exeter, Devon EX4 6AH.
The Natural Medicines Group, PO Box 5, Ilkeston, Derbyshire DE7 8LX.
The Register of Chinese Herbal Medicine, PO Box 400, Wembley, Middlesex HA9 9NZ.

USA
American Botanical Council, PO Box 210660, Austin, TX 78720.
American Herbal Products Association, PO Box 2410, PO Box 210660, Austin, TX 78720.
The American Herbalists' Guild, PO Box 1683, Soquel, CA 95073.
Northeast Herb Association, PO Box 266, Milton, NY 12547.
The Herb Research Federation, 1007 Pearl Street, Suite 500, Boulder CO 808302.

Australia
National Herbalists Association of Australia, Suite 14, 247–249 Kingsgrove Road, Kingsgrove, NSW 2208.

School of Herbal Medicine/Phytotherapy, PO Box 5310, Toowoomba, Queensland 4350.
Southern Cross Herbal School, PO Box 734, Gosford, NSW 2250.
Southern School of Natural Therapies, 43 Victoria Street, Fitzroy, Victoria 3065
Victorian Herbalists Association, 24 Russell Street, Northcote, Victoria 3070.

Canada
Ontario Herbalists Association, 7 Alpine Avenue, Toronto, ONT M6P 3R6.

Mail Order Herb Suppliers
G. Baldwin & Co, 171–74 Walworth Road, London SE17 1RW.
East West Herbs Ltd, Langston Piory Mews, Kingham, Oxon OX7 6UW.
Hambledon Herbs, Court Farm, Milverton, Somerset TA4 1NF.
Neal's Yard Remedies, 26–34 Ingate Place, London SW8 3NS.

Nurseries and Specialist Plant Suppliers
Cheshire Herbs, Fourfields, Forest Road, Little Budworth, Tarporeley, Cheshire CW6 9ES.
Chiltern Seeds, Bortree Stile, Ulverston, Cumbria LA12 7PB.
Iden Croft Herbs, Frittenden Road, Staplehurst, Kent TN12 0DN.
National Herb Centre, Banbury Road, Warmington, nr Banbury, Oxon OX17 1DF.
Poyntzfield Herb Nursery, Black Isle, By Dingwall, Ross & Cromarty IV7 8LX.

Suppliers
USA
Bay Laurel Farm, West Garzas Road, Camel Valley, CA 93924.
Frontier, Box 299, Norway, Iowa 52318.
May Way Trading Chinese Herb Company, 1338 Cypress Street, Oakland, CA 94607.
Herbs Products Co, 11012 Magnolia Blvd., North Hollywood, CA 91601.

Kiehls Pharmacy, 109 Third Avenue, New York, NY 10009.
Sage Mountain Herbs, PO Box 420, East Barre, VT 05649.

Australia
Australian Botanical Products Pty Ltd, 39 Melverton Drive, Hallam, Victoria 3803.
Blackmores Ltd, 23 Roseberry Street, Balgowlah, NSW 2093.
Greenridge Botanicals, PO Box 1197, Toowoomba Queensland 4350.
Essential Therapeutics, 6 Stuart Road, Lilydale, Victoria 3140.
Herbs of Gold Pty Ltd, 120 Milwood Avenue, Chatswood, NWS 2067.
Medi-Herb Pty Ltd, PO Box 713, Warwick, Queensland, 4370.
Southern Light Herbs, PO Box 227, Maldon, Victoria 3463.